TRACKING DOWN HIDDEN FOOD ALLERGY

By William G. Crook, M.D.
Illustrations by Cynthia P. Crook

ISBN 0-933478-05-4

Sixth Printing, 1985

Text © 1980, 1978 William G. Crook, M.D.
Illustrations © 1980, 1978 Cynthia Crook

PROFESSIONAL BOOKS • P.O. Box 3494 • Jackson, Tennessee 38303

This book is dedicated to Dr. William C. Deamer, Emeritus Professor of Pediatrics, University of California, San Francisco, whose perceptive observations and unselfish interest and encouragement have helped physicians all over the world suspect and identify hidden or delayed onset food allergies.

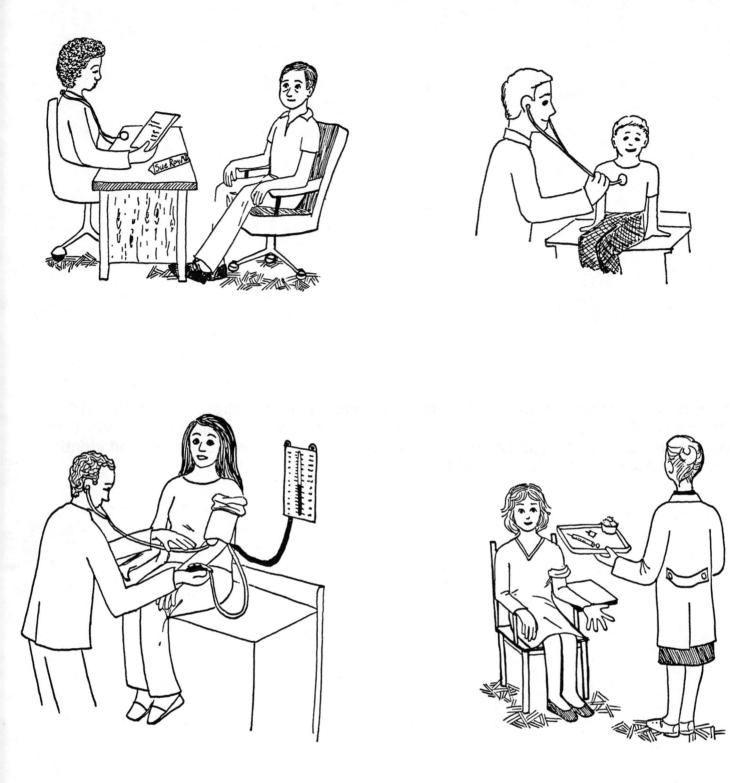

Before concluding that your symptoms are caused by an allergy, go to your physician for a careful history and physical examination, and appropriate laboratory studies or tests. Here's why such an examination is important: Many other disorders can cause similar symptoms.

However, if a careful check-up shows no apparent physical disease or other obvious cause for the symptoms described in this book, chances are they're caused by a hidden food allergy.

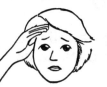
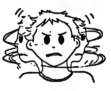

WHAT THIS BOOK IS ALL ABOUT

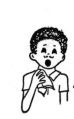

If you or your child are bothered by fatigue, headache, drowsiness, irritability, hyperactivity (or other nervous system symptoms), recurring ear problems, dark circles under your eyes, pallor (in the absence of anemia), wheezing, coughing, recurring abdominal pain, muscle aching, urinary symptoms, and persistent nasal congestion, go to your doctor for a careful check-up, including a history and physical examination, complete blood count, urinalysis and tuberculin test. Your physician may also feel that a chest x-ray, thyroid tests and other blood studies are necessary.

But before undergoing more complex, expensive and painful tests or procedures, including gastrointestinal x-rays, urinary tract x-rays, electroencephalographic examinations and brain scans, psychiatric evaluation or surgery, try an elimination diet and see if your symptoms get better.

Also, try an elimination diet before you settle for symptomatic relief with tranquilizers, mood elevators or other drugs which may help some of your symptoms without getting at their cause.

This book is written for both adults and children. *And it gives specific instructions for carrying out elimination diets, which will let you know whether or not your symptoms are caused by adverse or allergic reactions to foods you're eating every day.*

On pages 11-23, you'll find pictures and food lists which will help you know what foods you can and cannot eat on Elimination Diet A—a diet which avoids foods which commonly cause hidden allergies in Americans (milk, corn, wheat, egg, chocolate, citrus, beet & cane sugar, coffee, and tea); Diet A also avoids food dyes, flavors, additives and alcoholic beverages.

On page 24, you'll find shopping tips which tell you where to obtain the foods you need for Elimination Diet A (on page 40 you'll find further shopping tips).

On pages 25-37, you'll find food lists, illustrations and menus for Elimination Diet B (sometimes called the Rare Food or "Cave Man" Diet). **In carrying out this diet, avoid any and every food you eat more than once a week.**

On pages 41 and 42, you'll find a list of food sources which will help you or your food store obtain foods you'll need for your diet.

On pages 43-55, you'll find questions and answers which will help you prepare menus and obtain the cooperation of other family members.

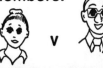

v

You'll also find instructions which will help you keep accurate records and which tell you **when and how to eliminate foods from your diet and when and how to add them back so as to find out if your symptoms are caused by foods you're eating.**

Although this question and answer section is adapted from a conversation between a physician and the mother of a child bothered by chronic health problems, you'll find that they're equally applicable to you, the adult allergy victim.

On pages 56-66, you'll find the story or parable of Timmy which illustrates the important concept of "allergic load." When your resistance is high and your load of allergy troublemakers is low, you're apt to remain symptom-free and well. Yet when your allergy trouble makers combine, they overcome your resistance and make you sick.

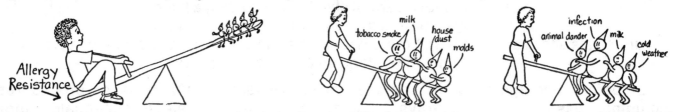

On pages 67-72, the parable, Susie's Cow's Milk Allergy, illustrates another important allergy principle which applies especially to hidden food allergy. Fortunately, even though you're allergic to a common food (such as milk, corn, or wheat) if you avoid the food for several months, your sensitivity to the food decreases (like a fire that dies down). So most allergy sufferers regain tolerance to a food they're allergic to if they avoid it for several months and then eat it in smaller amounts every 4 to 7 days.

A third parable on pages 73-75 tells you more about a rotated diet and gives you examples of such a diet.

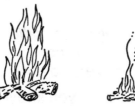

In tracking down a hidden food allergy, **you must keep careful records for several days before you start the diet. Then you'll need to continue your records during the period of elimination as well as when you're adding foods back.** This section, pages 78 & 79, gives you suggestions for accomplishing this goal.

You'll find a final children's story on pages 81-83, ("Helping Mary Stay on her Diet—The Diet Game.") It suggests a reward program to decrease "cheating" and increase compliance. You may want to try a similar plan and reward yourself for sticking with the diet and successfully completing it.

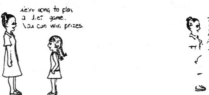

On pages 84-90, you'll find recipes you can use on Elimination Diet A and on pages 91-93, you'll find a short discussion of "the chemical problem," which troubles many people who suffer from food allergy.

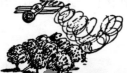

TABLE OF CONTENTS

WHAT IS ALLERGY?

The term "allergy" was coined in 1906 by Austrian pediatrician Clemens von Pirquet who put together two Greek words, allos (= other) and ergon (= work or action). *So an allergic person reacts to substances that don't bother other people.*

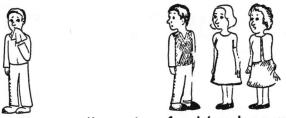

When you or your child develop an allergy to a food (such as milk), the food is called an *allergen.* Substances in your body which react with allergens are called *antibodies.*

When *allergens* and *antibodies* come together, reactions which occur resemble "tiny explosions." Histamine and other chemicals are released throughout the body. These chemicals (often called "mediators") make automatic muscles tighten up and go into spasm. And they cause blood vessels to leak fluid, and glands in the nose, bronchial tubes and other parts of the body to put out excessive mucus.

When you are highly sensitive to a food, such as strawberries or fish, the allergic reaction occurs rapidly . . . even violently . . . in a few seconds to a few minutes. Symptoms produced include rash, swelling, sneezing, wheezing, severe abdominal cramps, vomiting, and fainting. Such a reaction is termed an *obvious food allergy.* No elimination diets are needed to identify this sort of allergy.

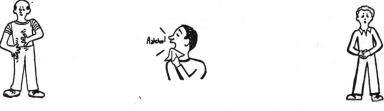

Many, many times more common is the type of allergy discussed in this book . . . *hidden food allergy.** This sort of allergy is also called "masked," "variable," or "delayed onset" food allergy.

Hidden food allergy is caused by foods you or your child eat daily, or several times a day. *The person with such an allergy tends to become allergic to his favorite foods.* And, strange as it may seem, he's apt to be addicted to the foods making him sick. What's more, the food addict (like the cigarette or narcotic addict) may temporarily feel better after he takes in the substance he's addicted to. Accordingly, tracking down a hidden food allergy requires carefully planned and executed elimination diets. This book is designed to help you carry out such diets and to give you a clearer understanding of food allergy, how to recognize it, prevent it, and treat it.

---

*Four types of allergic reactions have been identified and classified. One of these (Type I) is mediated through a blood fraction called "IgE." Reactions of this type produce positive scratch tests in individuals sensitive to pollens and other inhalants, and much less commonly in individuals sensitive to food. However, most individuals who show the food reactions discussed in this book do *not* show positive scratch or other immunologic tests. And at this time (1980) the mechanism and explanation for such food reactions is unknown. Accordingly many immunologists and other physicians prefer to call these food reactions "intolerances" or "hypersensitivities" or "adverse reactions."

ACKNOWLEDGEMENTS

The instructions in this book are based on the concepts of many pioneer food allergists, including Dr. Theron Randolph, and the late Doctors Albert Rowe and Herbert Rinkel.

I am grateful to these physicians and to many others whose observations have contributed to my understanding of hidden food allergy . . . especially Doctors James Breneman, Clifford Brooks, William Deamer, Lawrence Dickey, Benjamin Feingold, Hobart Feldman, John Gerrard, Jerome Glaser, Douglas Heiner, Stephen Lockey, John Maclennan, Marshall Mandell, Tatsuo Matsumura, Joseph Miller, Joseph Morgan, James O'Shea, Guy Pfeiffer, Doris Rapp, Albert Rowe, Jr., Douglas Sandberg, Frederic Speer, Francis Waickman, Robert Owen and James Willoughby.

Particular thanks are due to a number of these individuals, as well as to Dr. Robert Collier, Dr. David Eubank, Stella Fitts, Margo Galloway-Brown, Marjorie Howe, Sherry Hudson, Nell Sellers, Alice Spragins and Marion Winbush, all of whom reviewed the manuscript for this book and made helpful suggestions for improving it. And, finally, I appreciate the untiring work of Georgia Deaton who typed it, and Janet Berger and Patrick Youngblood who put it all together.

TRACKING DOWN HIDDEN FOOD ALLERGY

You Can Suspect A Hidden Food Allergy When You or Your Child...

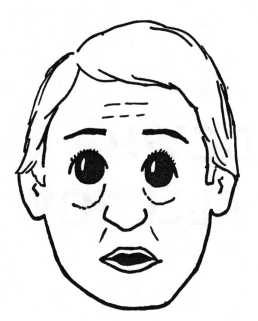

develop dark circles or "bags" under your eyes,

sniff, snort, clear your throat or push your nose up.

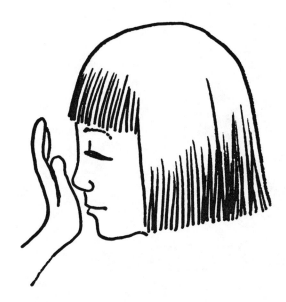

are nervous,
irritable or
overactive

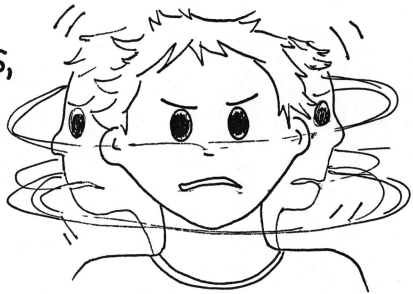

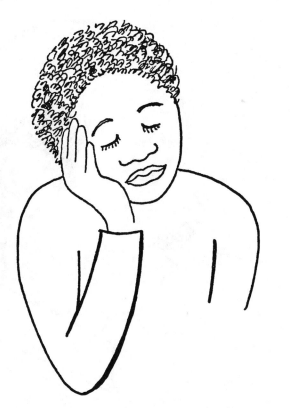

or tired,
droopy
and drowsy

5

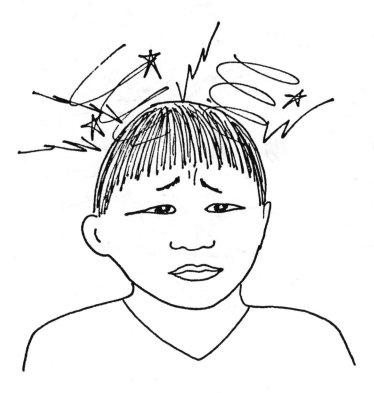

complain of
headache,
stomachache
or muscle
aches.

are bothered
by coughing
or wheezing.

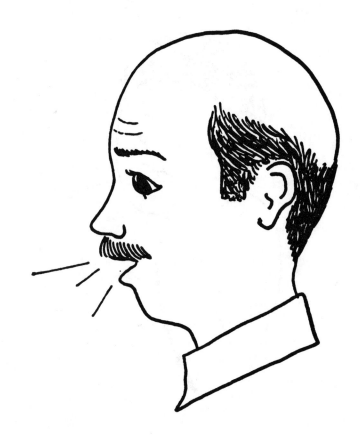

were plagued by irritability and frequent digestive and respiratory problems in infancy and/or early childhood.

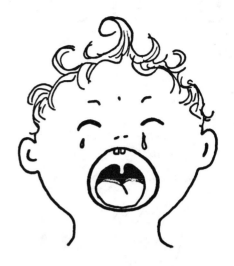

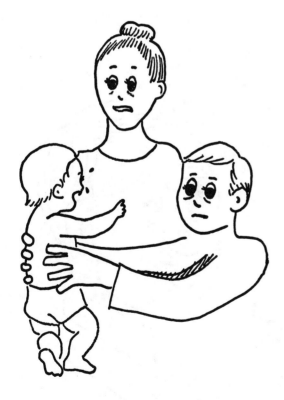

... or other members of your family are bothered by allergies

You're Probably Asking...

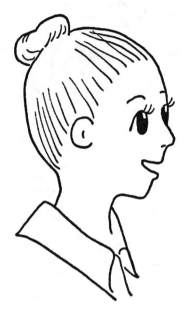

"How do I find out if my symptoms are caused by something I eat?"

"You carry out an elimination diet avoiding some or all of your favorite foods."

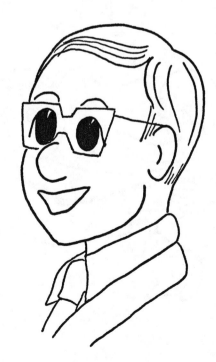

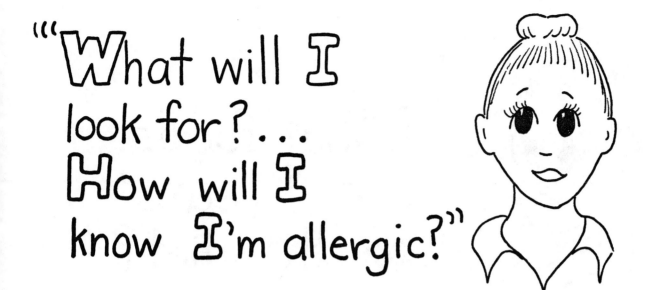

"What will I look for?... How will I know I'm allergic?"

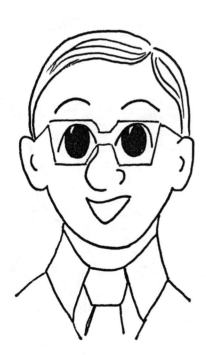

"If you're allergic to the foods you avoid, your symptoms will improve or disappear. And they will return when you eat the foods again."

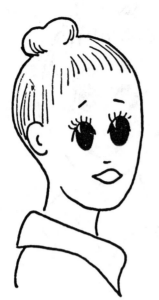

"What foods can I eat on the diet?"

"There are two diets. We nearly always start with Diet A. Later on, we may need to use Diet B."

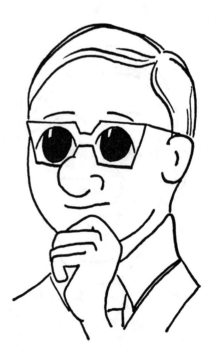

ELIMINATION
DIET A

Elimination Diet A
Foods You or Your Child Can Eat

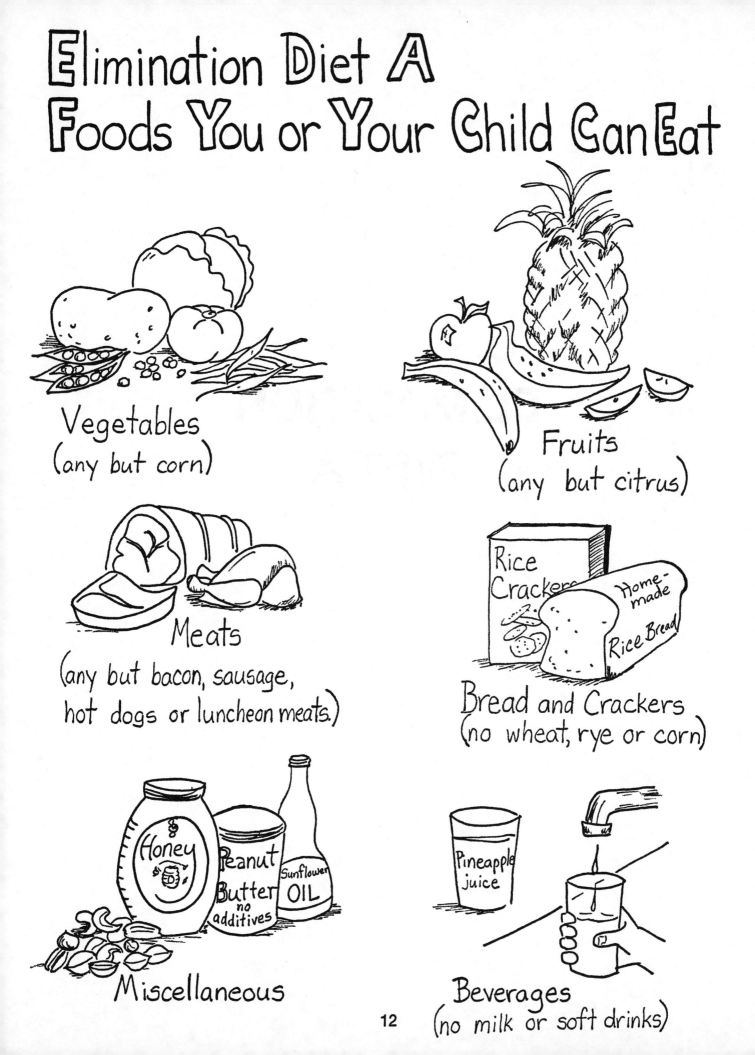

Vegetables
(any but corn)

Fruits
(any but citrus)

Meats
(any but bacon, sausage,
hot dogs or luncheon meats.)

Rice Crackers

Home-made

Rice Bread

Bread and Crackers
(no wheat, rye or corn)

Honey

Peanut Butter
no additives

Sunflower OIL

Miscellaneous

Pineapple juice

Beverages
(no milk or soft drinks)

Vegetables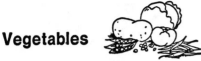

White potatoes
Green peas, beans and
  other legumes
Tomatoes
Sweet potatoes
Cabbage
Lettuce
Carrots
Squash
Asparagus, cauliflower,
Onions, radishes, beets,
Celery, green peppers,
Greens (beet, mustard,
spinach, etc.), cucum-
bers, okra, egg plant,
Brussel sprouts, turnips,
Kale, avocado, broccoli,
Mushrooms, parsnips,
Collards, rutabaga

Fruits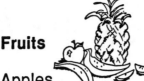

Apples
Bananas
Grapes
Peaches
Pears
Pineapple
Prunes
Raisins
Cantaloupe
Watermelon
Strawberries
Figs, dates, cherries
Apricots, coconut, plums,
Nectarines, persimmons,
Blackberries, blueberries,
Cranberries, dewberries,
Boysenberries, raspber-
ries, loganberries

Meats

Beef
Chicken
Pork
Veal
Turkey
Lamb
Fish (trout, salmon,
  tuna, sardines, etc.)
Clams, lobster, crab,
Oysters, shrimp,
Squirrel, rabbit,
Quail, duck, goose,
Game birds, pheasant

Bread & Crackers:

You'll usually need to bake your own bread*, since most commercial products contain wheat. You can use oat, rice, potato, starch, arrowroot, or soy flours.
Rice crackers & cakes**

Beverages:

Water, pineapple juice, grape juice, apple juice.

Miscellaneous:

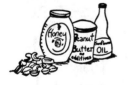

Nuts . . . Peanuts, cashews, pistachios, English walnuts, black walnuts, hickory nuts, pecans, butternuts, almonds, Brazil nuts, chestnuts, hazel nuts.
Honey, pure maple syrup, peanut butter**
Safflower oil, sunflower oil, Willow Run margarine**

―――――――
*See Recipes, page 87 & 89.
**See Shopping Tips, page 40.

Foods You or Your Child Must Avoid

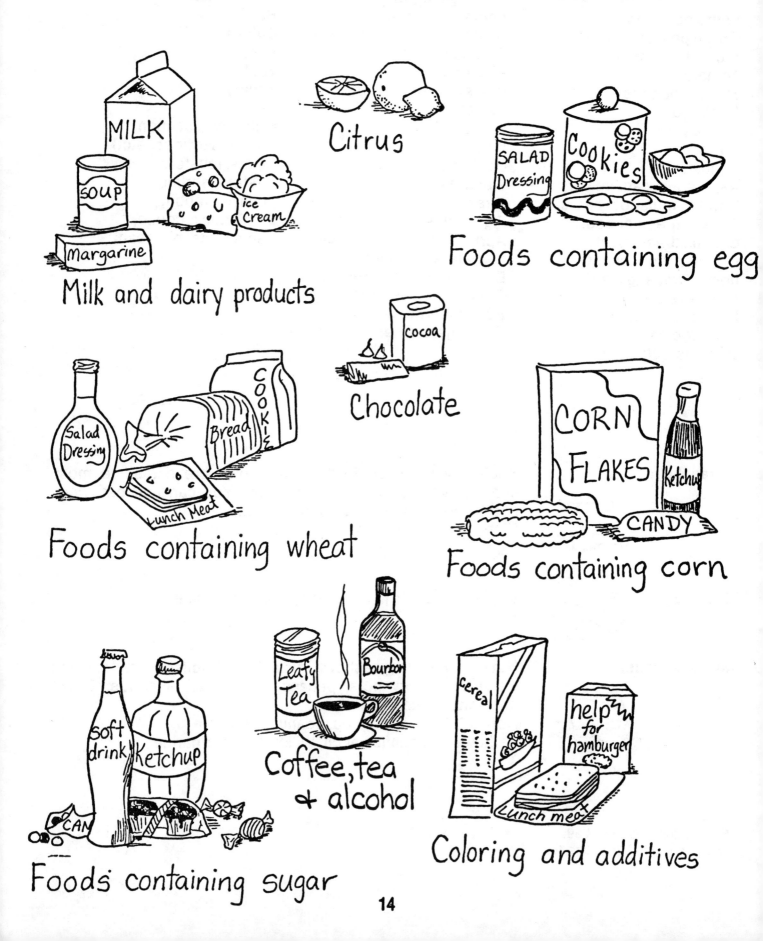

MILK
SOUP
ice Cream
margarine
Milk and dairy products

Citrus

SALAD Dressing
Cookies
Foods containing egg

cocoa
Chocolate

Salad Dressing
Bread
COOKIES
Lunch Meat
Foods containing wheat

CORN FLAKES
Ketchup
CANDY
Foods containing corn

soft drink
Ketchup
CAN
Foods containing sugar

Leafy Tea
Bourbon
Coffee, tea & alcohol

Cereal
help for hamburger
Lunch meat
Coloring and additives

Milk-containing foods:

Cheese, butter, ice cream, margarines, breads, soups, cookies, candies, luncheon meats and other manufactured or processed foods.

Egg-containing foods:

Cakes, cookies, ice cream, pies, macaroni, salad dressings, noodles, pancake mixes and other manufactured or processed foods.

Wheat-containing foods:

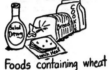

Foods containing wheat

Breads, cookies, crackers, soups, cereals, candies, batters, luncheon meats, pancake mixes, salad dressings, gravies, and other commercially prepared foods.

Corn-containing foods:

Foods containing corn

Candies, breads, pastries, batters, cereals, ketchup, peanut butter, bacon, and many other processed and refined products which contain corn oils, starches or sugars.

Sugar-containing foods:

Candies, soft drinks, cookies, ice cream, salad dressings, ketchup, and countless other packaged and processed foods.

Chocolate-& *Cola*-containing foods:

Chocolate

Candies, snack foods, cereals, desserts.

Orange- & *citrus*-containing foods:

Citrus

Oranges, limes, grapefruit, Sprite, flavorings in desserts, and other processed foods.

Coffee, tea & alcohol:

Coffee, tea & alcohol

All coffee and tea (including instant and caffein free) products must be avoided. Also all alcoholic beverages.

Foods containing *coloring, flavoring & additives:*

Processed & packaged foods, including cereals, soft drinks, ketchup, mustard, hot dogs, luncheon meats, and many others.

NOTE:
To lessen your chances of making mistakes in planning, shopping and carrying out an elimination diet, avoid packaged and processed foods wherever possible. And when you use such foods, READ LABELS. Also try to avoid canned foods since many cans are lined with phenolic resins which cause symptoms in chemically sensitive individuals.

Suggestions for Breakfast

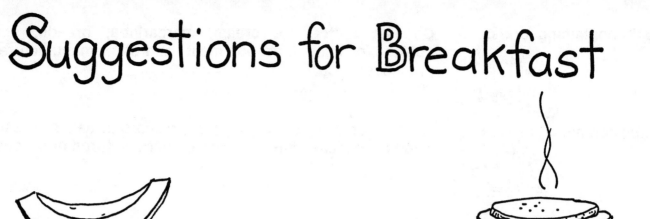

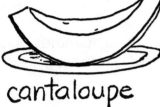

cantaloupe

special pancakes

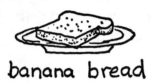

banana bread

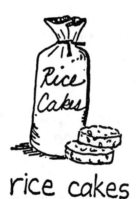

strawberries

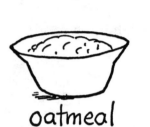

oatmeal

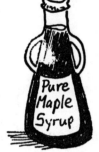

maple syrup

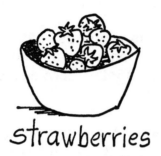

rice cakes

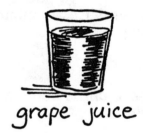

grape juice

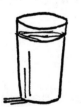

pineapple juice

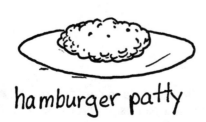

hamburger patty

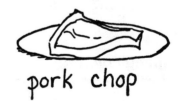

pork chop

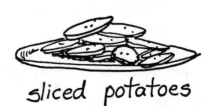

sliced potatoes

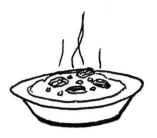

Hot oatmeal (Quaker rolled oats), topped with shredded nuts or raisins
Sweeten with maple syrup, or honey.
Use Jolly Joan Soyquik flavored with honey & vanilla bean.
Banana, or stewed prunes.
Apple juice.
Banana bread.

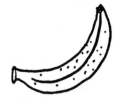

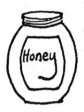

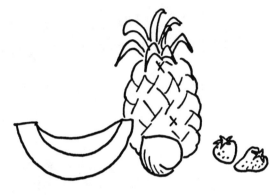

Cantaloupe
Special pancakes (made with grainless mix or rice flour*)
Honey, maple syrup, pecans
Grape juice

Fresh peaches or strawberries, with honey
Fish (bake or fry in safflower oil using rice flour* for batter).
Sprinkle with almonds

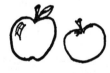

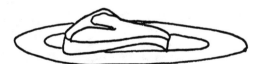

Pork chops
Potatoes (sliced, and cooked in safflower oil)*
Pineapple juice
Peaches, grapes, strawberries or other permitted fruit (no oranges)
Honey, or pure maple syrup
Rice cakes or crackers*

Sliced apples (or other permitted fruit)
Ground beef (3 oz. or more)
Rice cakes*
Pure maple syrup, or honey
Welch's grape juice

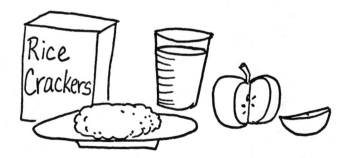

*See pages 40 & 41.

Ideas For Lunch

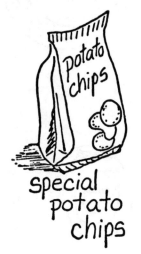

special
potato
chips

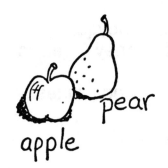

pear

apple

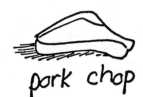

peanut butter and
honey on rice crackers

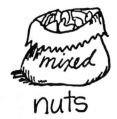

nuts

baked chicken

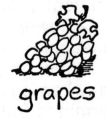

Celery sticks

banana treat

pork chop

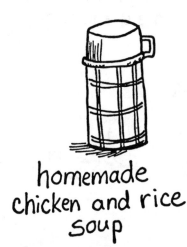

homemade
chicken and rice
soup

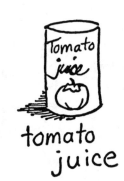

tomato
juice

grapes

Hamburger patty, salt &
pepper (no buns or "fixings")
Banana treat (banana, spread
with peanut butter, put halves
together, drizzle with honey
and roll in ground peanuts)
Carrot sticks
Peanuts
Rice crackers**
Pineapple juice

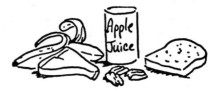

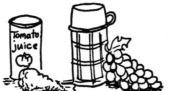

Pork chop
Banana
English walnuts
Banana bread*
Apple juice

Homemake chicken and rice
soup*,
Rice crackers
Grapes or other fresh fruit
Chicken leg baked or fried in
rice batter
Tomato juice

Tuna fish (water-packed) on
rice crackers, or taken in a
small container
Potato chips (made with
safflower or cottonseed
oil) which contain no
additives**
Plums or other fresh fruit
Pecans
Grape juice

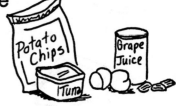

Peanut butter and honey on
rice crackers
Celery sticks
Almonds
Apple (or other fresh fruit)
Apple juice (unsweetened)

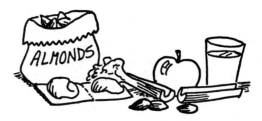

---

*See recipes, pp. 85-90.
**See pp. 40-41.

Suggestions for Supper

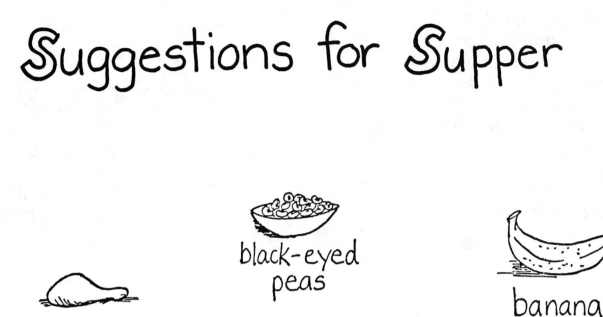

black-eyed peas

banana

chicken

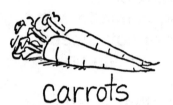

carrots

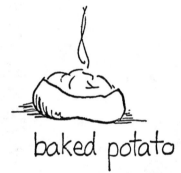

baked potato

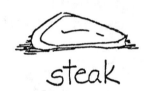

steak

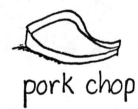

pork chop

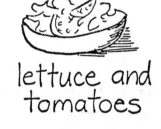

lettuce and tomatoes

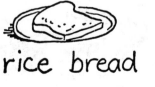

rice bread

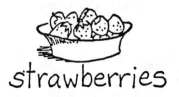

strawberries

Hamburger patty
French fried potatoes (use safflower oil)
Willow Run margarine
Green peas
Lettuce & tomato salad
Sliced pineapple (in own juice)
Rice crackers or cakes
Special boiled mayonnaise*

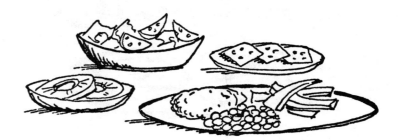

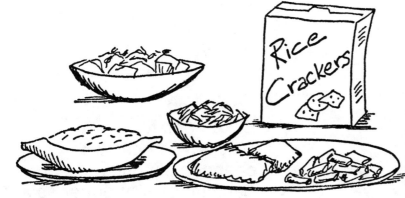

Fish (bake or fry in safflower oil, using rice flour for batter)
Green beans
Sweet potato
Rice crackers
Cole slaw*
Dessert . . . mixed fruits covered with shredded coconut

*See Recipes, page 86.

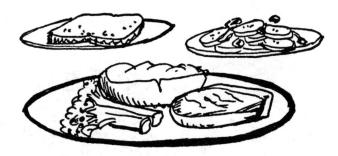

Steak
Baked potato
Broccoli
Rice bread
Willow Run margarine
Dessert . . . sliced bananas
chopped pecans, honey

Oven-baked chicken
Baked sweet potato
Willow Run margarine
Carrots
Banana bread
Apple-nut-raisin salad on
lettuce leaf
Strawberries and honey

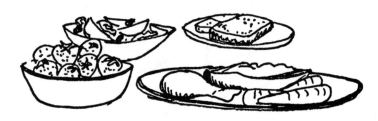

Pork chop
Baked potato
Black-eyed peas with
chopped almonds
Banana, peanut butter salad*
Banana bread*
Watermelon, cantaloupe (or
other fruit)

*See Recipes pg. 87, 89.

Snacks—
At Work or After School

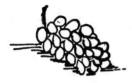

grapes

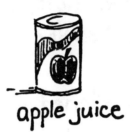

apple juice

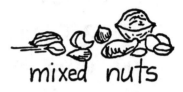

mixed nuts

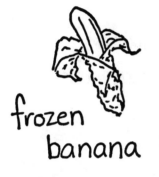

frozen
banana

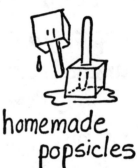

homemade
popsicles

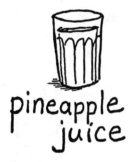

pineapple
juice

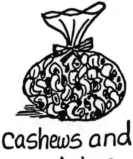

cashews and
raisins

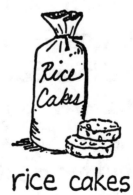

rice cakes

fresh fruits

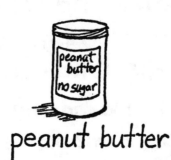

peanut butter

Shopping Tips for Elimination Diet A

FROM YOUR SUPERMARKET:

1. Stock up on all fresh fruits and vegetables (except corn and citrus fruits).

2. Buy chicken, beef, pork and fish including tuna canned in spring water. (Stay away from hot dogs, bacon, sausage, ham & luncheon meats since these products usually contain coloring & additives.)

3. Buy pure unsweetened juices including apple, grape, pineapple & tomato (no orange or grapefruit.)

4. Other suggestions: sugar & additive-free peanut butter, additive-free potato chips (should not contain corn oil), Quaker Rolled Oats, pineapple or other fruit packed in its own juice & coconut (in shell).

FROM YOUR HEALTH FOOD STORE:

1. Hain Sunflower or Safflower oil
2. Nuts in shell or additive-free nuts.
3. Chico-San or Arden Rice Cakes
4. Other suggestions include EnerG Rice Flour & EnerG Egg Replacer, local honey, sugar-free peanut butter, Health Valley Potato Chips, Sonoma dried fruits, Willow Run margarine, steel cut oats brown rice and pure maple syrup.

ELIMINATION
DIET B

(ALSO KNOWN AS THE RARE FOOD OR CAVE MAN DIET)

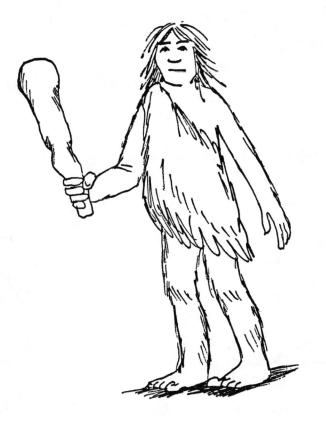

Elimination Diet B
Foods You or Your Child Can Eat

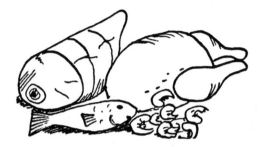

Meats
(any but beef, chicken and pork)

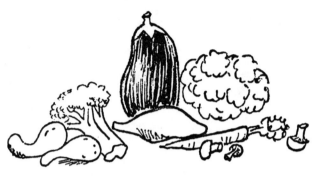

Vegetables
(any but corn, irish potato and legume

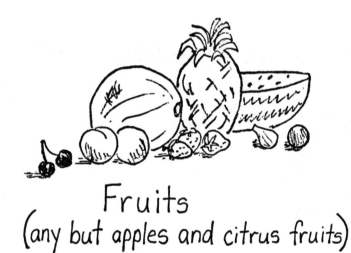

Fruits
(any but apples and citrus fruits)

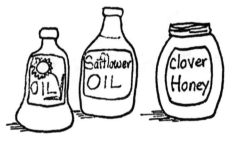

Safflower or Sunflower Oil
and Honey

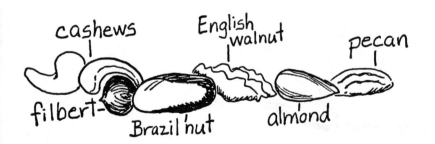

cashews

English walnut

pecan

filbert-

Brazil nut

almond

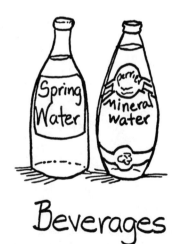

Beverages

Vegetables

Sweet potatoes
Cabbage
Carrots
Squash
Asparagus
Cauliflower
Celery
Okra
Onions
Radishes
Greens (beet, mustard,
    spinach, etc.)
Cucumbers
Egg plant
Brussel sprouts
Kale
Avocado
Broccoli
Parsnips
Collards
Rutabaga

Fruits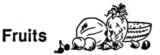

Bananas*
Grapes*
Peaches
Pears
Pineapple
Prunes
Mangos
Cantaloupe
Watermelon
Strawberries
Figs
Dates
Cherries
Apricots
Coconut
Plums
Persimmons
Blackberries
Blueberries
Cranberries
Dewberries
Raspberries
Loganberries

Meats (or Substitutes)

Turkey**
Fish
Lamb
Shrimp
Deer
Rabbit
Duck
Goose
Oysters
Clams
Lobster
Crab
Squirrel
Pheasant
Frog legs
Quail

Breads, Cakes, Crackers: Because wheat, corn, rice, rye, oats, barley and other grains are common causes of chronic allergy, and because all grains belong to the same "food family," *avoid all grains while on this diet.* (This means your child eats no bread, crackers, cakes and cookies while on Diet B.*)

Beverages: Bottled mineral water or spring water.

Miscellaneous: Nuts . . . cashews, pistachios, English walnuts, black walnuts, hickory nuts, pecans, butternuts, almonds, Brazil nuts, chestnuts, hazel nuts. *(No peanuts.)*

Clover honey (or similar locally produced honey), pure maple syrup.

Safflower and sunflower oils.

---

*The purpose of Diet B is to avoid any and every food you or your child eats more than once a week. Accordingly, if you love bananas, eliminate them. And if you snack regularly on grapes, eliminate them too.
**Many commercial turkeys are basted with milk, corn or other additives and must be avoided on Elimination Diet B.

Foods You or Your Child Must Avoid

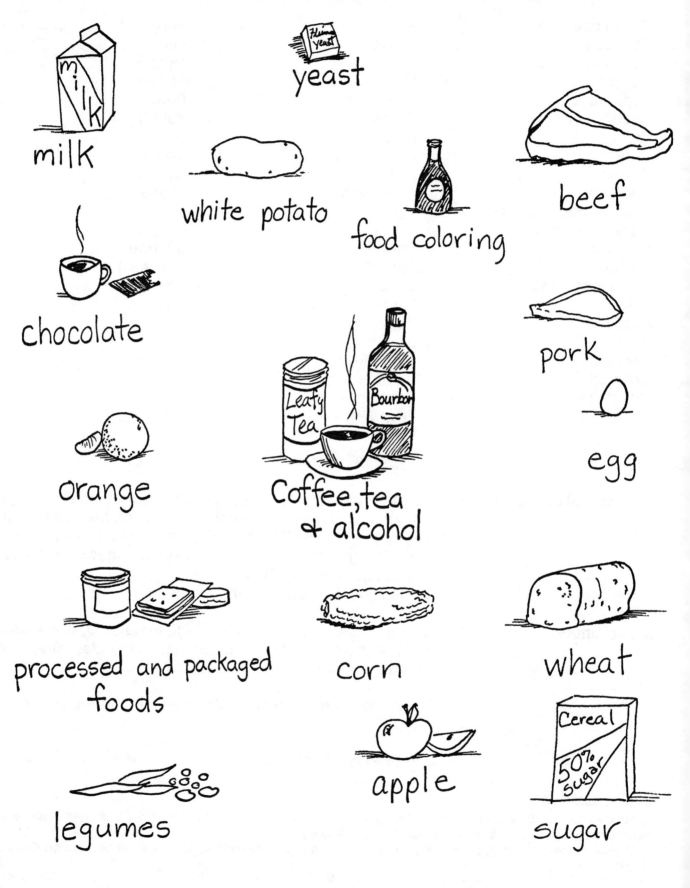

milk

yeast

beef

white potato

food coloring

chocolate

pork

orange

Coffee, tea & alcohol

egg

processed and packaged foods

corn

wheat

apple

legumes

sugar

Milk-containing foods:

Milk and dairy products, including cheese, butter, ice cream, margarines, and yogurt, cream soups, breads, crackers, cookies, cakes, candies, luncheon meats, and other manufactured or processed foods.

Egg-containing foods:

Egg or any foods containing egg, including custards, cakes, cookies, ice cream, pies, macaroni, salad dressings, noodles, pancake mixes, and other manufactured or processed foods.

Grain-containing foods:

Wheat, corn, rye, barley, rice, and all other grains or foods containing grains. This includes all breads, cookies, crackers, cereals, batters, luncheon meats, pancake mixes, candies and a wide variety of other packaged and processed foods.

Citrus:

Orange, grapefruit, lemon, and all foods containing citrus fruits or citric acid.

Sugar-containing foods:

Cane and beet sugars, including candies, cakes, sugar-coated cereals, ice cream, carbonated beverages, and a wide variety of processed and packaged foods which contain sugar.

Legumes:

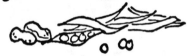

Peanuts, beans and peas of all kinds, including string beans, lima beans, soy beans, baked beans, green peas, field peas and black-eyed peas. Soy bean protein ("textured protein") is also hidden in a wide variety of manufactured foods.

Chocolate & Cola-containing foods:

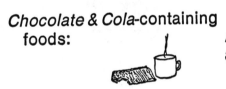

Avoid chocolate and cola drinks of all kinds; also all candies and other foods to which chocolate has been added.

Meats:

All forms of beef, pork and chicken, including luncheon meats, hot dogs, bacon, sausage and hamburger.

Fruits & Vegetables:

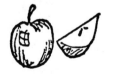

White potato, including baked potatoes, french fried potatoes, potato chips and any other food containing potato; corn, rice, apple (including fresh, frozen or dried apples, apple juice or any foods containing apple flavoring); and any fruit or vegetable eaten more often than once a week.

Yeast-containing foods:

Breads, wine, vinegar, mushrooms, vitamins, condiments, dried fruits and many stored, frozen or canned foods including fruit juices.

Coffee, tea & alcohol:

All coffee and tea (including instant and caffein free) products must be avoided. Also all alcoholic beverages.

29

Suggestions for Breakfast

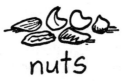

nuts

lamburger

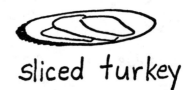

fresh melon

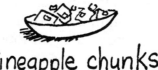

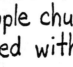

pineapple chunks
sprinkled with pecans

sweet potato slices
cooked in safflower oil

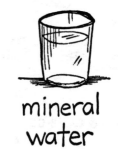

mineral
water

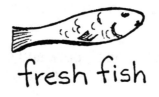

fresh fish

sliced turkey

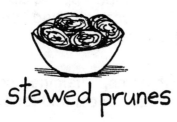

stewed prunes

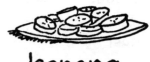

banana

Lamb patty
Sliced bananas
Chopped pecans
Honey
Bottled mineral water

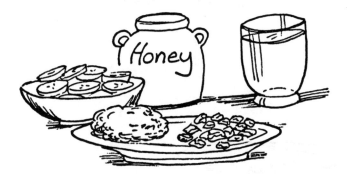

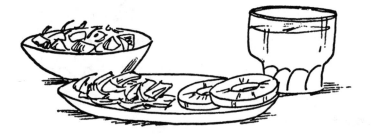

Fresh fish cooked in
safflower oil
Fresh pineapple
Shredded fresh coconut &
chopped Brazil nuts
Bottled mineral water

Turkey slices
Sweet potato slices (cooked
in safflower oil)
Stewed prunes or fresh melon
Chopped cashew nuts
Bottled mineral water

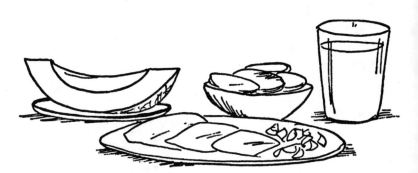

Ideas For Lunch

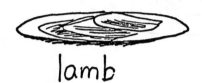

lamb

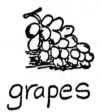

grapes

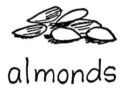

almonds

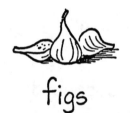

figs

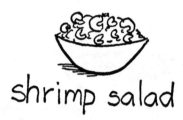

shrimp salad

raisins

pears

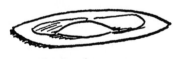

turkey

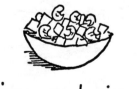

shrimp and pineapple

32

Slices of cold lamb
Banana treat (split banana,
spread with cashew nut
butter, put halves together,
drizzle with honey, and roll in
ground cashew nuts).
Bottled mineral water

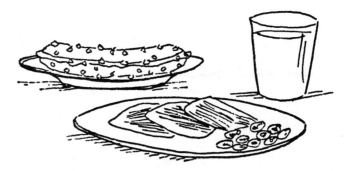

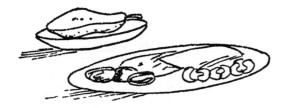

Turkey slices
Cashew nuts
Pear

Shrimp salad
made with chopped Brazil
nuts, chopped celery and
chopped raw carrots
Almonds
Grapes

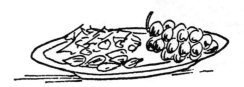

Suggestions for Supper

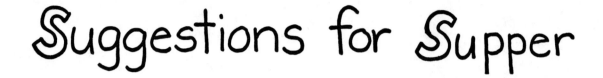

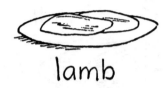
lamb

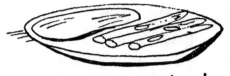
asparagus and almonds

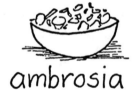
steamed carrots

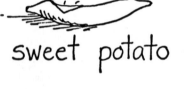
sweet potato

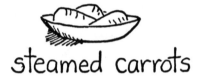
baked fish

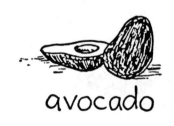
ambrosia

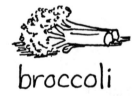
broccoli

avocado

banana

Broiled shrimp on skewers
with pineapple
Spinach
Baked squash
Fresh raspberries or other
allowable fruit in season

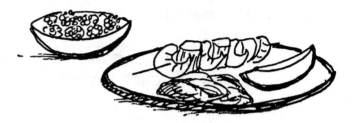

Roast duckling
Brussel sprouts
Celery and carrot sticks
Poached pears (core pears-
fill with chopped dates &
pecans and poach with equal
amounts of pure maple syrup
and water until tender)

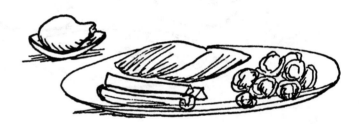

Pheasant
Baked potato
Vegetable medley, (saute
zucchini, shaved carrots &
onions in safflower oil)
Fruit salad (bananas &
grapes with shredded
coconut on top)

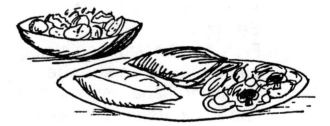

Turkey
Baked sweet potato
Cauliflower, baked, or fried in
safflower oil
Sea salt
Sliced bananas, honey, and
chopped English walnuts

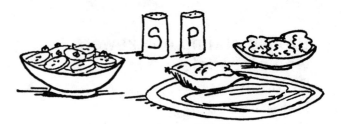

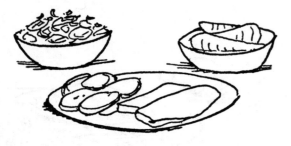

Fish, baked, or fried in
safflower oil
Squash (or other permitted
vegetable)
Boiled carrots
Sea salt
Ambrosia made with crushed
pineapple, fresh coconut and
pecans

Lamb
Asparagus & almonds
Sea salt
Fruit & nut salad, containing
pineapple, fresh strawberries
(or sliced bananas), coconut
and any nuts except peanuts.

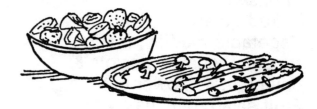

Snacks—
At Work or After School

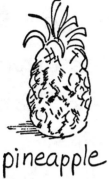
pineapple

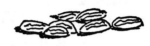
pecans

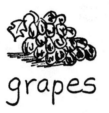
grapes

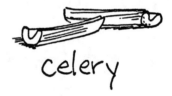
celery

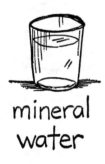
mineral water

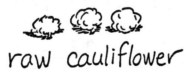
raw cauliflower

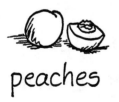
peaches

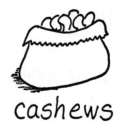
cashews

Shopping Tips for Elimination Diet B

From your supermarket:

1. Stock up on fresh fruits and vegetables which you do not usually eat such as asparagus, avocados, cherries, mangos, pears, pineapple, pomegranates, strawberries and sweet potatoes.

2. Buy lamb, fresh turkey, fresh fish, shrimp and other seafood.

3. Other suggestions: Nuts in shell including almonds, brazil nuts, coconut and pecans.

4. Bottled mineral water.

From your health food store:

1. Hain sunflower or safflower oil.

2. Nuts in shell or additive-free nuts.

3. Other suggestions: Pure maple syrup, bottled mineral water, local honey, cashew nut butter.

Other rare and exotic foods can be ordered from a variety of sources some of which are listed on pages 41 and 42.

MORE
SHOPPING TIPS
and
FOOD SOURCES

MORE SHOPPING TIPS*

1. Feature fresh foods.

2. Try to avoid canned, packaged and processed foods.

3. When using canned or packaged foods, READ LABELS CAREFULLY.

4. Avoid processed, smoked, or cured meats, such as salami, wieners, bacon, sausage, hotdogs, etc., since they often contain milk, corn, sugar, food coloring and other additives.

5. Avoid canned fruits packed in heavy or light syrup, since they contain cane or corn sugar. Instead, buy fruits packed in their own juices. Or, better still, use fresh fruits.

6. Some fish are canned in vegetable oil. Since the oil may be of unknown source, buy fresh fish or fish packed in water, or in its own oil.

7. Most commercially available nuts are roasted in vegetable oil and contain additives. Accordingly, buy nuts in the shell, or shelled nuts from a health food store.

8. Commercial peanut butter usually contains sugar. So use *pure* peanut butter (usually available from a health food store).

9. Most commercial frozen turkeys are basted with milk or corn. You'll need to avoid them and buy turkey from other sources.

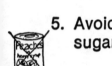

10. Use rice crackers for a bread substitute (read labels). Or you can bake your own bread using Ener-G rice flour*, or other special flour.

11. Use safflower oil in cooking or for salad dressings. (Combine with wine vinegar or apple cider vinegar).

12. Some commercial honeys come from sugar-fed bees. Such honey may cause symptoms in cane or beet sensitive children. Buy clover honey or other locally produced honey.

13. Willow Run margarine*, made from pure soybeans, can be found at most health food or specialty stores.

14. Unsweetened pineapple, apple, and Welch's grape juice are good substitutes for colas and other sweetened beverages. You can also freeze juices for homemade popsicles.**

15. Carob powder can be used as a substitute for chocolate.

16. Pure soy "milk" (made from Jolly Joan Soyquik) can be used as a milk substitute.***

17. Buy sea salt or canning salt, since some commercial salts contain corn starch.

---

*Some tips are appropriate for diet A while others are useful for diet B, and still others are helpful for both diets.
**See "Recipes", page 90.
***Soyquik may be flavored with vanilla bean and honey.

FOOD SOURCES

Cellu cereal-free baking powder
Cellu rice wafers, tapioca flour
Water packed fruits
Potato starch flour

Chicago Dietetic Supply, Inc.
LaGrange, Illinois 60525

Caracoa carob powder

El Molino Mills
City of Industry, California 91746

Rice cakes

Arden Organic
99 Pond Road
Asheville, North Carolina 28806

Imitation catsup (contains tomato paste,
water, honey, cider vinegar, sea salt
and natural spice).
Cashew butter

Hain Pure Food Company, Inc.
Los Angeles, California 90061

Rice crackers (contain whole brown rice,
sesame seeds & salt)

Chico San, Inc.
1144 West First Street
Chico, California 95926

Potato chips (contain potato, safflower
oil & salt. No additives).

Health Valley Natural Foods, Inc.
700 Union
Montebello, CA 90640

Sesame oil, safflower oil, sunflower
oil, peanut butter.

Arrowhead Mills, Inc.
Hereford, Texas 79045

Nuts & Seeds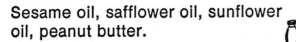

Midwest Nut & Seed Company, Inc.
1332 W. Grand
Chicago, Illinois 60622

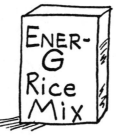

Ener-G rice mix
Ener-G egg replacer
Jolly Joan pure Soyquik

Ener-G Foods, Inc.
P.O. Box 24723
Seattle, Washington 98124

Unsweetened spreads
(raspberry, strawberry &
other fruits)

Westbrae Natural Foods
Berkeley, CA 94706

Rice Crunch Crackers, plain
(Kitanihon Company)

Tree of Life
P.O. Box 1391
St. Augustine, Florida 32084

Organic foods and exotic meats such
as game & game birds of the U.S.A., and
a few foreign animals

Czimer Food, Inc.
Rt. 1, Box 285
Lockport, Illinois 60441

Glass-canned natural Alaskan salmon
with no seasonings or preservatives

Briggs Way Company
Ugashik, Alaska 99683

Fresh & dried fruits

Lee's Fruit Company
P.O. Box 450, Hobby Hill
Leesburg, Florida 32748

Fresh fruits & vegetables

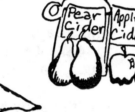

Vita Green Farms
P.O. Box 878, 1525 W. Vista Way
Vista, California 92083

Persimmons, zapota, cheramola,
prickly pear, avocado & pomegranate

Sam King
Alvarado Street
Fairmont, California 94530

Apples, pears, apple cider and
pear cider

Leslie Barnes
Kinagrow Farms
Belding, Michigan 48809

Sweet potatoes

Al Mueller
233 Dade Avenue
Ferguson, Missouri 63135

Fearn natural soya powder

Fearn Soya Foods
Melrose Park, Illinois 60160

Nuts, especially pecans

mixed nuts

J.H. O'Neal
P.O. Box 565
Donalsonville, Georgia 31745

Taro, mountain potato, yucca, boniata,
apio root, ginger and fresh fish

Del Farm Food Company
4610 N. Clark Street
Chicago, Illinois 60600

Bottled water, fruits and juices,
vegetables, baked goods, dairy
products, nuts, grains, honey,
flours, meats and seafoods

Shiloh Farms
Sulphur Springs, Arkansas 72768

Sonoma dried fruits

Timbercrest Farms
4791 Dry Creek Road
Healdsburg, California 95448

Also check with your local health food store. They may be able to supply some of the
foods on this list.

QUESTIONS
&
ANSWERS
ABOUT
ELIMINATION DIETS

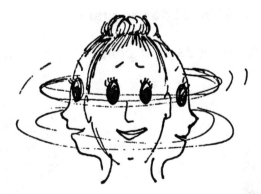

QUESTIONS AND ANSWERS
ABOUT
ELIMINATION DIETS*

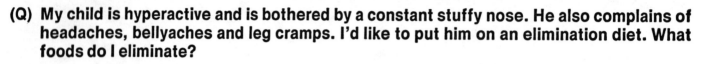

(Q) My child is hyperactive and is bothered by a constant stuffy nose. He also complains of headaches, bellyaches and leg cramps. I'd like to put him on an elimination diet. What foods do I eliminate?

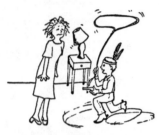

(A) You eliminate his favorite foods. Here's why: The more of a food a child eats, the greater his chances are of developing an allergy to the food. To make things easier for you, I've prepared two diets. The first of these, DIET A (see page 12) eliminates foods* many Americans eat every day including:

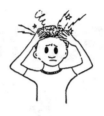

- Milk (and all dairy products)
- Egg
- Wheat
- Corn
- Cane and beet sugar
- Orange (and other citrus fruits)
- Chocolate
- Food coloring and additives

If your child's symptoms don't improve on Diet A, let him resume his usual diet for a few days, then try Diet B.

(Q) How do I get started on Diet A? What do I do first?

(A) *Prepare menus and purchase foods your child will eat while on the diet. This requires careful planning.*

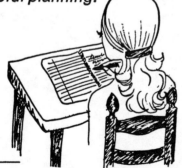

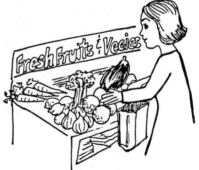

*Although this question and answer section is adapted from a tape-recorded conversation between a physician and the parent of a child with suspected food allergies, the instructions apply equally to adults. Adults should also eliminate coffee, tea and alcoholic beverages.

Try to avoid commercially prepared or manufactured foods. Here's why: Such foods often contain sugar, wheat, milk, corn, food coloring, additives and other "hidden" ingredients which may be responsible for your child's symptoms.

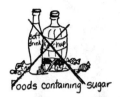
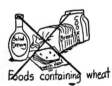
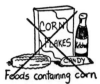
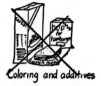

Discuss the diet with your child. (See "Diet Reward Program," page 82.) Emphasize the foods he *can* eat rather than telling him what he *can't* eat. Study the list of permitted foods and feature those you know he'll like.

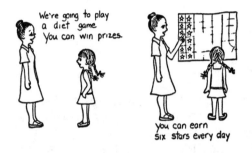

Get the help of your spouse and the cooperation of grandparents, brothers, sisters, aunts, uncles, baby sitters, neighbors, teachers and other school and nursery personnel.

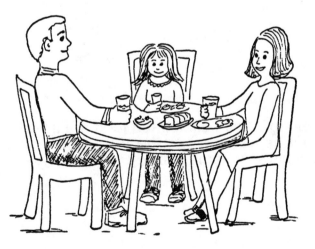

(Q) Tell me more about the diet.

(A) The diet is divided into two different parts:

Part 1: You eliminate foods to see if your child's symptoms improve or disappear.

Part 2: You return foods to the diet . . . one at a time . . . and note which foods cause symptoms to return.

(Q) How will I know the diet is really making a difference?

(A) By keeping a record of your child's symptoms:

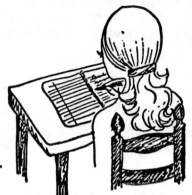

a. For 3 days before beginning the diet.
b. While he's on the diet (7 days, sometimes longer).
c. While you're adding foods (8 days, sometimes longer).

(See "Symptoms and Diet Diary," page 78).

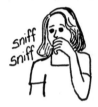

(Q) How will he feel on the diet?

(A) During the first 2 to 4 days of the diet, he's apt to feel irritable. He may become more hyperactive or more tired and droopy. He may develop a headache or leg cramps. And he may be "mad" at you (and the world) because he isn't getting foods he craves, especially sweets. (He may act like a two-pack-a-day smoker who's just given up the "weed". Children and adults who suffer from a hidden food allergy are often addicted to foods they're allergic to.)

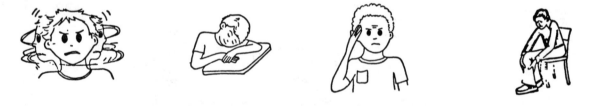

Usually, if your child is allergic to an eliminated food, he'll feel better by the 4th, 5th or 6th day. And almost always he'll improve by the 10th day. Occasionally, though, it'll take two to three weeks before his symptoms subside completely.

(Q) If he improves on the diet, what do I do then? When and how do I return foods to his diet?

(A) *After you're certain your child's symptoms have improved, and the improvement has continued for at least 2 days, begin adding foods . . . one food at a time. If your child is allergic to one or more of the eliminated foods, he should develop symptoms when he eats the foods again.*

(Q) When I add a food, does it make any difference what form the food is in?

(A) *Yes. Yes. Yes.* Add the food in *pure* form. For example, when you give your child wheat, use Cream-O-Wheat rather than bread, since bread contains milk and other ingredients. If you're adding milk, use whole milk rather than ice cream, since ice cream contains sugar, corn syrup and other ingredients.

Here are suggestions for returning foods to your child's diet:

Citrus: Peel an orange and let your child eat it. You can also offer him fresh orange juice. Canned or frozen orange juice without sugar is OK, but fresh fruit is better.

Wheat: Use Cream-O-Wheat breakfast cereal. Prepare as directed. Add honey or salt if you wish. Or use the special milk substitute, Soyquik* (prepared from soybeans). If he doesn't like it, try covering the cereal with banana plus a little pineapple juice (you can mix them together in a blender).

If your child won't eat the Cream-O-Wheat, you can give him bite-sized shredded wheat. (However, the shredded wheat contains the additive BHT which occasionally may cause symptoms. So a pure wheat product without additives is better.)

Egg: Give him a soft or hard-boiled egg, or eggs scrambled or fried in safflower or sunflower oil.

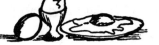

Chocolate: Use pure Baker's cooking chocolate or Hershey's cocoa powder. Add honey.

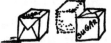

Milk: Use whole milk. Or make a pineapple or banana milkshake in your blender.

Corn: Use fresh corn on the cob, or canned corn. Or offer him popcorn (prepared at home and popped with safflower or sunflower oil), corn syrup, grits or hominy.

Sugar: Use plain cane sugar. (You might turn your child loose on a box of sugar lumps.) Or you can add sugar to apple, grape or pineapple juice. (If you use beet sugar at your house, challenge with it, too.)

Food Coloring: Buy a set of McCormick's or French's food dyes and colors. Put ½ teaspoonful of each color in a glass. Add 1 teaspoonful of the mixture to pineapple or grape juice and let him drink all he wants.

*See page 41.

think I understand what you want me to do. However, a few points aren't clear. Please repeat your instructions.

(A) OK. Here they are:

1. *Keep your child on the diet until you're absolutely certain his symptoms improve, and this improvement continues for at least 2 days.* This usually takes about 7 days (occasionally a day or two less). However, some children with chronic food allergy won't improve until they've been on the diet for 10 to 14 days. And in an occasional child, it'll take up to 21 days.

2. If your child fails to improve after following the diet for 14 days, "turn him loose." Let him eat what he wants. If his symptoms worsen (such as headache, hyperactivity or stuffiness), chances are one or more foods bother him. And you'll have to do further dietary detective work to find the troublemakers.

 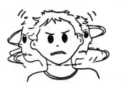 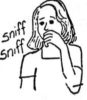

3. If your child improves on the diet, return the eliminated foods, *one at a time*, and see if he develops any symptoms. Here's how you go about it: . . . .

a. *Add, first, the food you least suspect, and save the food you most suspect until last. Remember, your child is apt to be allergic to his favorite foods.*

b. If you have no particular suspects, here's a suggested way of returning foods to your child's diet:

    1st day—orange
    2nd day—wheat
    3rd day—egg
    4th day—food coloring
    5th day—chocolate
    6th day—corn
    7th day—sugar
    8th day—milk

4. Give your child all he wants of the eliminated food for breakfast. If he shows no reaction, give him more of the food for lunch and supper (and in-between meals, too).

5. *Keep the rest of his diet the same.* This is important, so I'll give you an example: Suppose you return orange to his diet on the first day and he shows no reaction. Does this mean you can continue to give him an orange? NO. *He gets orange only on the day of challenge and he doesn't get orange again until all foods have been added, one at a time, and the entire diet testing has been completed.*

---

*If a person's symptoms are caused by a hidden food allergy and he improves after eliminating the food for 5-10 days, *the symptoms will nearly always return on the first day the food is eaten again.* However in some individuals symptoms may not return until the food is eaten in quantity for several consecutive days. Moreover *if a food trouble maker is eliminated from a person's diet for 2 or 3 weeks or longer, he will usually regain some tolerance to the food and larger quantities must be consumed for several consecutive days before symptoms reappear.* (See also the parable, Susie's Cow's Milk Allergy, page 68.)

6. If he shows no symptoms after adding a food the first day, add another food the second day in exactly the same way, giving him all he wants, *unless he shows a reaction.*

7. If you think he develops symptoms when you add a food, but aren't certain, give him more of the food until the symptoms are obvious.

8. If your child shows an obvious reaction after eating a food (such as stuffiness, cough, irritability, hyperactivity, drowsiness, headache, stomachache or flushing), don't give more of that food. *Wait until the reactions subside (usually 24 to 48 hours) before you add another food.*

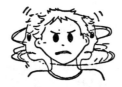

If the reaction really bothers him, you can usually shorten it by giving him 1 teaspoonful of "soda mixture" (2 parts baking soda and 1 part potassium bicarbonate), or by giving him Alka Seltzer Gold* dissolved in a half-glass water (2 tablets for teenagers and adults; 1 tablet for children 6 to 12; ½ tablet for children 1 to 5). A laxative such as milk of magnesia will also help terminate the reaction by more rapidly removing the offending food from the intestinal tract.

(Q) I hope I won't have to do Diet B, but tell me about it anyway in case I do.

(A) I call Diet B the "Rare Food" or "Cave Man" diet. In addition to the foods you eliminate on Diet A, you'll need to avoid peanuts, soy (and other members of the pea-bean family of foods), pork, beef, chicken, white potato, tomato, rice, oatmeal, *and any other food your child eats more than once a week.*

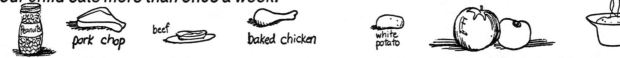

For example, if your child eats bananas every day, add bananas to the list of foods you eliminate. And if he snacks on pecans, avoid them. But if your child *rarely* eats a food, you need *not* omit it.

(Q) My goodness, this is a strange diet. Won't he starve?

(A) This diet *is* different. However, it's supposed to be. Because *our purpose in prescribing Diet B is to avoid foods your child usually eats.*** But as difficult as this diet seems to be, you'll be offering your child a variety of wholesome foods. (See list on page 27.) Do you think you can do it?

(Q) I suppose so . . . I can do anything I have to do. But let me repeat your instructions so I can be certain I understand them.

---

*Alka Seltzer in gold foil *without aspirin.*
**For older children and adults with severe and incapacitating allergies, a number of physicians have adopted an even more comprehensive elimination diet program. This program begins with a 4 or 5 day fast. While fasting, the patient consumes spring water only. Then after symptoms subside, foods are added 4 times a day for the next two weeks and reactions are noted, just as they are on Diets A & B. Such fasting is usually (but not always) carried out in a hospital.

I feel Diet A hasn't given me the answers I'm looking for, I'll try Diet B. On this diet, I eliminate the 8 Diet A foods plus peas, beans, peanuts, soy, pork, beef, chicken, potato, rice, oatmeal, and *any other food my child eats more than once a week.* So I'll be eliminating 15 to 20 foods.

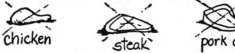

chicken   steak   pork chop   rice bread

(A) That's right.

(Q) How about returning these foods to the diet? Do I proceed as I did . . . adding only one food a day?

(A) That's one way to do it. However, it would take you 3 or 4 weeks to complete the diet . . .

(Q) That's a long time. And it would be hard for me to hold my child in line and keep him from cheating. Is there another way to do Diet B in less time?

(A) Yes. Carry out the elimination phase of the diet until your child's symptoms improve, just as we've already discussed. However, if your child improves promptly (as, for example, in 4 or 5 days), begin adding foods sooner.

You can also shorten the diet by adding three foods each day.

(Q) How would I do this? Please explain.

(A) Add a food (such as orange) for breakfast. If no reaction occurs*, introduce a second food (such as beef) at lunch. If no reaction occurs add a third food (such as potato) for supper.

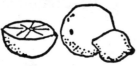

The following day add 3 more foods. And so on. This will reduce the "adding back" phase of the diet from 3 weeks to about 7 to 10 days.

(Q) Would that work as well?

baked potato

(A) Perhaps. And such a rapid addition of foods would have its advantages. One of them would be completing Diet B in much less time . . . two weeks rather than three or more weeks. Another advantage relates to one of the peculiarities of a "hidden" food allergy.

(Q) Could you explain?

(A) I'll try. If a person avoids a food he's allergic to for a week and then eats it again, it'll nearly always cause a reaction. But if he avoids it for two or more weeks, the level of his allergy may die down* so he may show little reaction when he eats it again, especially if he consumes only a small amount.

*See footnote page 48 and "Susie's Cow's Milk Allergy," page 68.

(Q) From what you've told me, I believe it'll be best for me to add one food each meal. Will that be OK?

(A) Yes. I believe this will be the easiest and best way for you.

(Q) OK. Now that's settled, I'd like your suggestions for getting my child to cooperate and stay on the diet.

(A) Plan the diet carefully. Discuss it with your child ahead of time. Purchase and feature foods he'll like. Don't force him to eat foods he's never liked. Don't worry if his diet is limited. Even if he loses a pound or two, it won't hurt him, he'll soon catch up.

Plan "The Diet Reward Game" carefully so he'll have something to look forward to each day. (See page 82.).

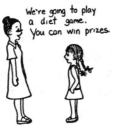

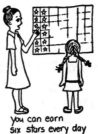

Most important of all, have other family members follow the same diet. If older children or your husband insist on desserts or other foods not on the diet, don't serve them at the table. Instead, wait until the dieting child has gone to bed.

(Q) Can he follow the diet and still go to school?

(A) Possibly . . . if you're sure your child will cooperate and won't cheat. Obviously, you'll have to prepare his school lunches at home. However, when you return foods to his diet, it may be wise to keep him at home. Then you can be sure he stays on the diet . . . more important, you can see reactions when he eats foods he's allergic to.

(Q) Is it best to start with Diet A? Or would you recommend going ahead with Diet B? Doing Diet B first might save me time and trouble.*

(A) That's true. And I sometimes recommend Diet B first. However, I usually recommend Diet A to begin with. Here's why:

1. Most food-sensitive children will improve on Diet A.

2. Diet A is easier than Diet B, because you can feed your child ground beef patties, steak, pork chops, chicken, Irish potatoes and apples . . . foods which most children like. So he'll be more apt to cooperate with you.

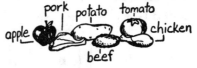

3. The rest of your family can easily eat the same diet. This will make things easier.

---

*Adults with severe or long lasting health problems caused by hidden food allergies may be allergic to many, many foods. Accordingly, such adults will be more apt to find help by following Diet B.

(Q) When, why and under what circumstances will it be necessary to try Diet B?

(A) This will depend on a lot of things. So I'll make a few comments. Although the foods which most commonly cause allergic reactions in my patients are milk, sugar, corn, wheat, egg, chocolate, orange and food coloring, other foods can also cause trouble.

So even if your child improves when you remove milk, corn, wheat, egg, sugar, chocolate or food coloring from his diet, he may continue to show symptoms because of allergy to beef, pork, chicken, apple and potato (or other foods). *And the only way you can tell if these foods bother your child is to eliminate them from his diet and see if his symptoms improve.* Then you let him eat the foods again and see if his symptoms return.

(Q) All right. I think I understand. But to make sure, let me repeat your instructions. You want me to do Elimination Diet A for 7 to 10 days, keeping a record of my child's symptoms for 3 days before I start the diet, as well as for the week or so he's on the diet. Then, after I'm sure his symptoms are better, I add the foods, one at a time, to see which foods bother him and which foods do not. And I continue my records.

(A) That's right.

(Q) Suppose I complete the diet and note obvious reactions with a couple of foods. Yet there are other foods I'm not sure about . . . what do I do then?

(A) Keep the foods which caused definite reactions out of the diet indefinitely. And re-test the foods you're uncertain about. Here's how you can do it:

Let him eat the suspected food several days in a row, such as Friday, Saturday, Sunday, Monday and Tuesday. Eliminate it on Wednesday, Thursday, Friday, Saturday and Sunday. Then load him up with the food on Monday. If he's allergic to it, he should develop symptoms. If he shows no symptoms, chances are he isn't allergic to that food.

(Q) I think I understand . . . but suppose Johnny shows a reaction when he eats wheat or egg . . . or when he drinks milk. Does this mean he'll always be allergic to these foods?

(A) Yes. To some degree. And his symptoms will nearly always return if he consumes as much of a food as he did before you put him on his diet.

However, if your child avoids a food he's allergic to for several months, he usually regains some tolerance to it. And he may not develop symptoms unless he eats it several days in a row.*

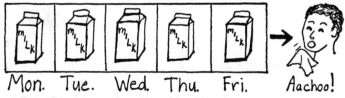

_____
*See "Susie's Cow's Milk Allergy," page 68.

(Q) How do I find out?

(A) By trial and error.

(Q) I'm not sure I understand . . . please explain.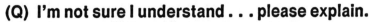

(A) I'll do my best. When a child avoids a food he's allergic to for several months, he'll generally lose some of his allergy to the food (like a fire that dies down).

For example, if your child is bothered by hyperactivity, stuffed up nose, headache and stomachache while drinking a quart of milk a day, he may be able to eat an occasional ice cream cone or cheese and cracker sandwich after he's eliminated milk from his diet for several months.

However, suppose he eats a dish of ice cream or a piece of cheese, or drinks a glass of milk after he has avoided them for a couple of months, and he shows no reaction. In such a situation, you may say to yourself, "Johnny drank a glass of milk and it didn't bother him, so maybe he isn't allergic to milk after all."

But if you start giving him milk every day, within a few days some of his symptoms will return. And before you know it, he'll develop the same health problems he had before you took him off the milk.

(Q) I think this point is clear, but why does a food bother a child on some occasions and not on others? For example, I've heard of milk allergic children who "kept a cold" all winter and who cleared up when they stopped drinking milk. Yet, they could drink milk in the summertime without symptoms. Why?

(A) I don't really know. However, along with many other physicians interested in food allergy, I've found that many allergic children can eat foods in the summer they can't eat in the winter.

Part of the problem may be chilling. Yet, some of the child's difficulties may be caused by wintertime furnaces, especially in colder weather. At such times, furnaces are turned on more often and cause more air turbulence. This stirs up dust and mold spores in the air and dries out the child's respiratory membranes. And all of these factors tend to make him more susceptible to wintertime infections.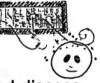

In addition, during the winter, the child spends more time in the house and disease-producing germs are more prevalent. So the combination of cold weather, cold germs, dust and other household inhalants, added to a food allergy, causes many children to develop health problems during the winter.*

---

*See "Timmy and the Allergy See Saw," page 58.

(Q) Do other allergies, such as hayfever due to grass or bronchitis due to dust and smoke, have anything to do with the amount of an allergy-causing food a child can eat?

(A) Yes. The more allergy troublemakers your child is exposed to, the greater are his chances of developing an allergic illness. For example, let's suppose your child is allergic to milk, corn, chocolate, spring grasses and house dust. (Yet, he isn't *severely* allergic to any one of these substances.)

Accordingly, he may play ball in the spring without being bothered by hayfever. And he may be able to eat an occasional piece of cornbread or chocolate birthday cake without symptoms.

But if he eats a sack of popcorn, a candy bar, and drinks a glass of chocolate milk all in the same day (after cutting the grass), he may become irritable, nervous and hyperactive. What's more, all these things together may make him develop an attack of asthma.

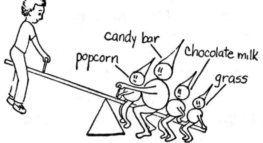

(Q) I'm beginning to understand more about hidden food allergy. But suppose my child is allergic to egg and I keep him off egg for 3 months. Then I feed him an egg for breakfast and it doesn't bother him. How will I know how much and how often I can feed him egg in the future?*

(A) I'm glad you asked. It'll give me a chance to talk about a rotated diet.**
Physicians interested in hidden food allergy have found that their allergic patients who rotate their diets usually get along well and develop fewer new food allergies.

Rotating the diet means eating a food only once every 4 to 7 days. For example, if you find your child is allergic to egg, and, after avoiding it for several months, he eats an egg and it doesn't bother him, you can try giving him egg once a week and see if he tolerates it. You can do the same with other foods.

S	M	T	W	T	F	S
1	2	**3**	4	5	6	7
8	9	**10**	11	12	13	**14**
15	16	**17**	18	19	20	21
22	23	**24**	25	26	27	28
29	30	**31**				

⌐ EGG DAY

(Q) Aren't some foods "kin" to each other . . . like chicken and egg, wheat and corn, or milk and beef? And is a person who is allergic to one food more apt to become sensitive to another food in the same "family"?

---

*See "Susie's Cow's Milk Allergy," page 68.
**See "Rotated Diets," page 74 & 75.

54

(A) The answer to both of your questions is "yes." Foods are "kin" to each other. Commonly known food families include the grain family, the citrus family, and the legume family (peas, peanuts, beans and soybeans). And while there are many exceptions, people who are sensitive to one food in a family are more apt to be sensitive . . . or to become sensitive . . . to another food in the same family.

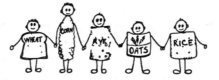

I've found that wheat-sensitive patients are especially apt to become sensitive to corn or rye. So, in such patients, I'm apt to say, "You'd be smart not to go overboard eating cornbread. And if you eat rye bread every day, you're almost certain to develop an allergy to rye."

While on the subject of grains, I'll say a word about rice and oats. Although your child can eat these grains on Diet A, if you find your child is allergic to any grain, experiment further with his diet to see if rice, oats or other grains cause trouble.

Now for a word on milk and hamburgers. Most milk-sensitive children eat hamburgers without reaction. However, because cow's milk and hamburger come from the same animal, if your child is allergic to milk, try him off beef for a week, then add it back and see what happens. And if your child is allergic to egg, I'd suggest you offer him chicken only once every 4 to 7 days.

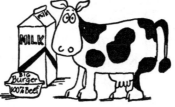

. . . Is there anything else you'd like to know? Anything at all?

(Q) Nothing I can think of at the moment. But my head is spinning. Do you have further suggestions?

(A) Read, review and study all of the instructions I've given you. And when you've finished you'll find that tracking down a hidden food allergy will be easier than you think it'll be.

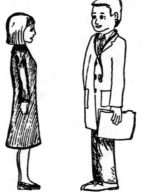

Physicians can find a comprehensive discussion of food families in the Frederic Speer's book, Food Allergy (PSG Publishing Co., Inc., Littleton , Mass. 1978) and food allergy patients can obtain additional information from The Cookbook/Guide To Eating For Allergy by Virginia Nichols (3550 Fair Oaks Drive, Xenia, Ohio 45385).

PARABLES ABOUT ALLERGY

Confucius say, "A journey of a thousand miles starts with one step." And overcoming your allergies, like the journey Confucius was talking about, requires many steps. Maybe not a thousand. But many.

And Dr. Susan Dees of Duke University, in talking about allergies some years ago, said in effect, "The more the allergic person knows about himself and the things he's sensitive to, and the more he knows about allergies and how they affect him, the better are his chances of overcoming them."

To help you understand more about allergies, especially food allergies, study the parables you'll find in the next 20 pages. Each one illustrates one or more important principles about allergy.

This first parable about Timmy and the allergy see-saw helps you understand the concept of "allergic load". Your allergic symptoms may be caused by many different substances ("gremlins"), including foods, pollens, house dust, molds, and animal danders.

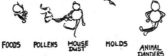

FOODS POLLENS HOUSE DUST MOLDS ANIMAL DANDERS

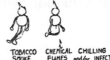

TOBACCO SMOKE CHEMICAL FUMES and/or CHILLING INFECTION

In addition, you may be sensitive to tobacco smoke and chemical fumes which increase your allergic load. Finally, chilling and infection may also increase your chances of developing allergic symptoms.

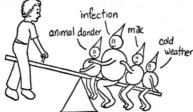

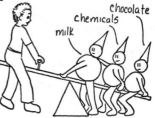

If you understand the story of Timmy and his allergy see-saw and identify your allergy troublemakers ("gremlins") and keep them under control, you'll have a better chance of staying well.

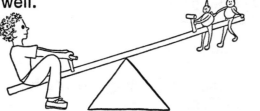

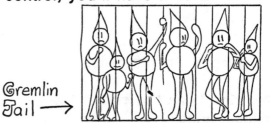

Gremlin Jail →

The second parable, "Susie's Cow's Milk Allergy" illustrates several important principles you'll need to know about hidden or delayed onset food allergy. Here they are:

(a) Hidden food allergies are caused by foods you eat every day. When you eliminate them, your symptoms will usually clear up within a week. (b) Then if you eat the foods again *following this short period of elimination,* your symptoms will return. (c) However, if you eliminate a food trouble maker for several months, you'll usually regain some tolerance to the food. (d) After regaining tolerance, you can eat the food occasionally (such as every 4 to 7 days) without causing symptoms. (e) Yet if you eat a lot of the food every day, your tolerance will break down and your symptoms will return.

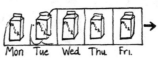

Mon Tue Wed Thu Fri.

The third parable, "How Paco's Mother Controls Food Allergy Gremlins" briefly tells you about rotated diets, and if you've developed an allergy to one or more foods you'll lessen your chances of becoming allergic to other foods by varying or rotating your diet.

THE STORY
OF
TIMMY

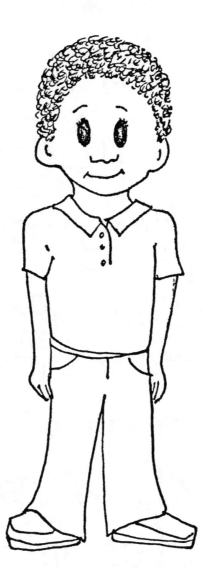

The Story of Timmy and the Allergy See-saw

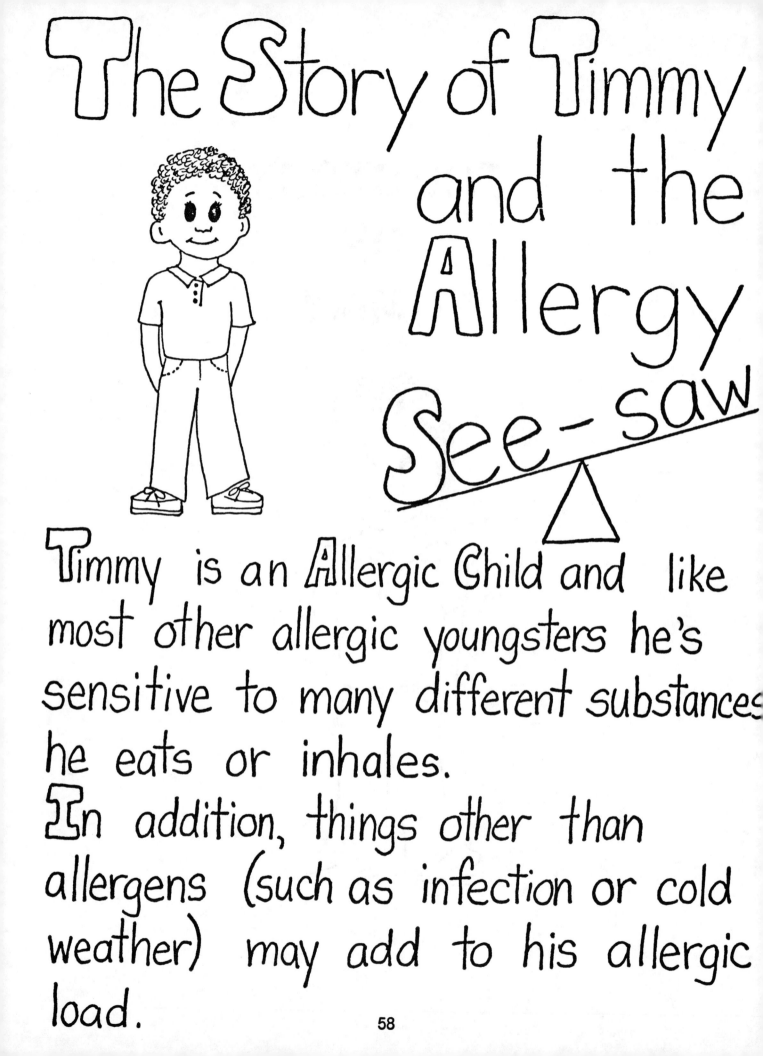

Timmy is an Allergic Child and like most other allergic youngsters he's sensitive to many different substances he eats or inhales.

In addition, things other than allergens (such as infection or cold weather) may add to his allergic load.

58

We'll call these trouble-makers

"GREMLINS"

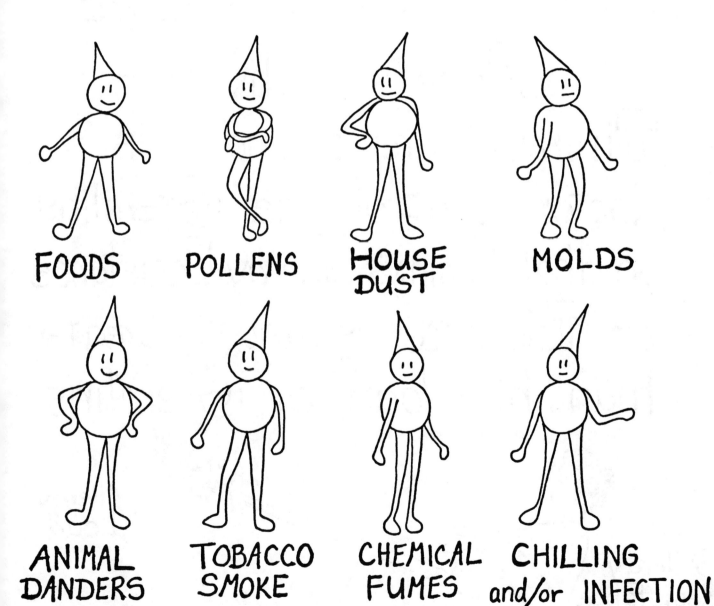

FOODS POLLENS HOUSE DUST MOLDS

ANIMAL DANDERS TOBACCO SMOKE CHEMICAL FUMES CHILLING and/or INFECTION

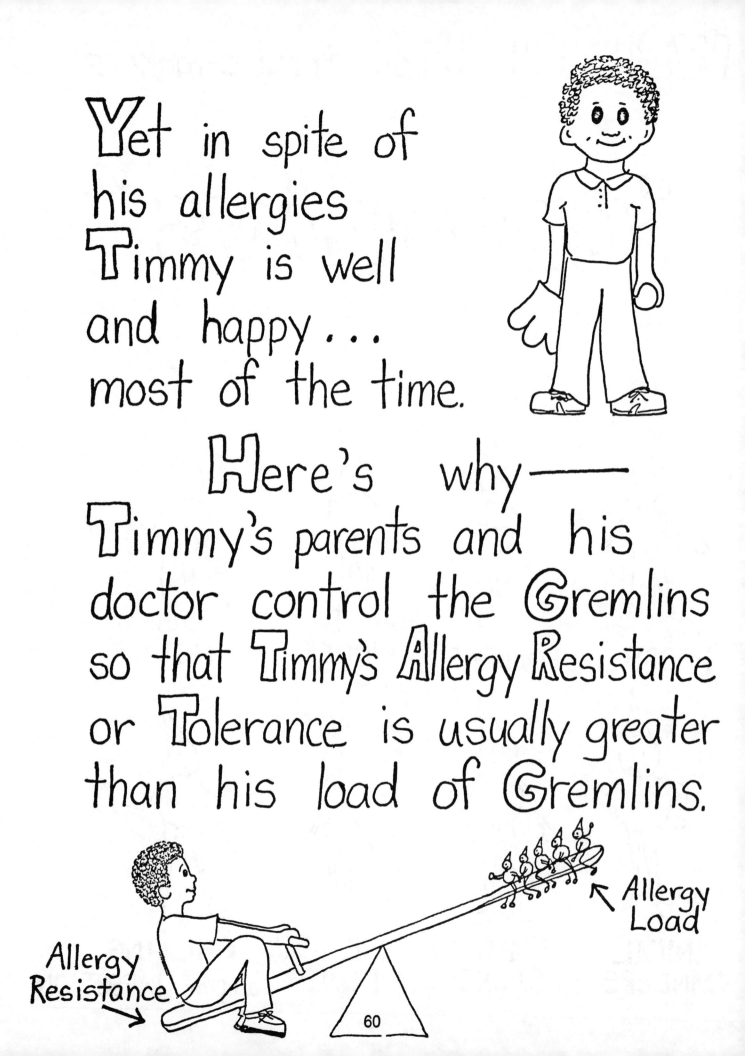

Yet in spite of his allergies Timmy is well and happy... most of the time.

Here's why— Timmy's parents and his doctor control the Gremlins so that Timmy's Allergy Resistance or Tolerance is usually greater than his load of Gremlins.

Allergy Load

Allergy Resistance

Here are examples—
Although Timmy is allergic
to milk, he
can drink an
occasional glass
or eat ice cream at a birthday
party without getting sick.

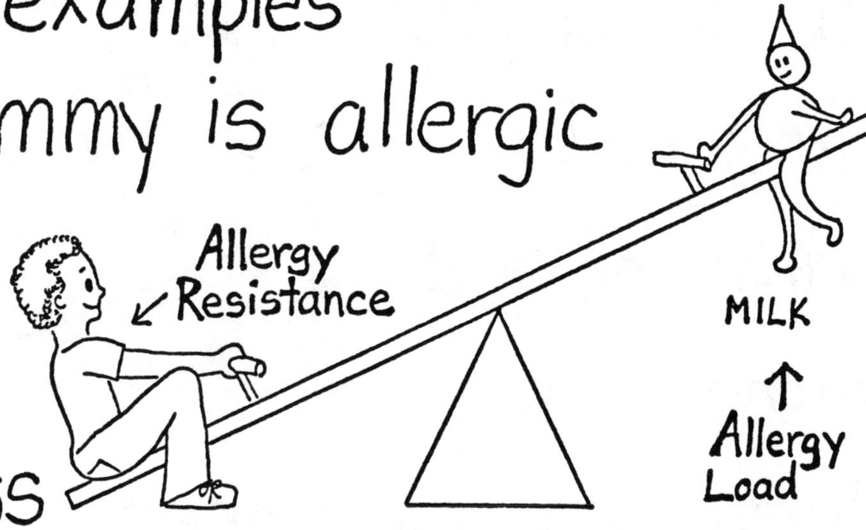

Allergy
Resistance

MILK

Allergy
Load

And Timmy can go through
the ragweed season
with few
symptoms
if he stays
away from milk
and doesn't play in a
field full of ragweed.

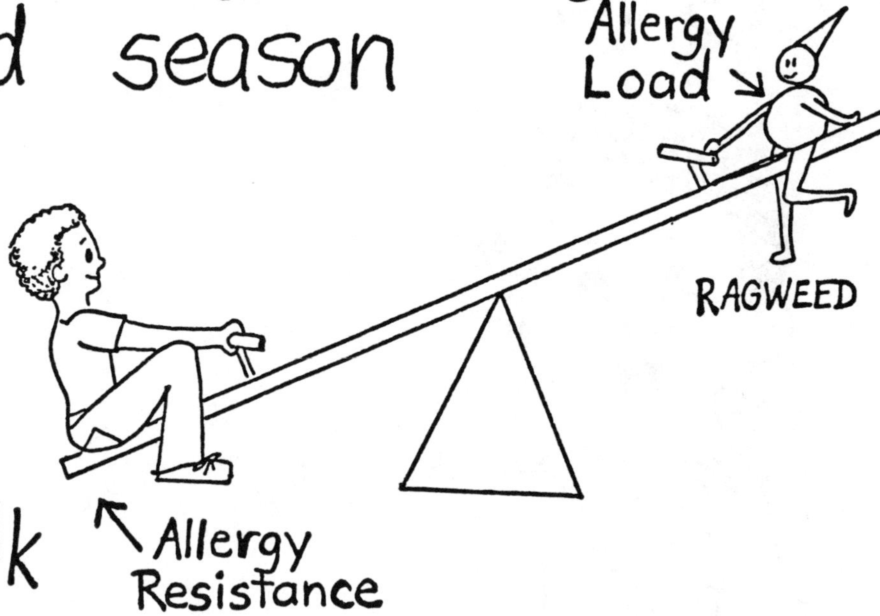

Allergy
Load

RAGWEED

Allergy
Resistance

But if Timmy drinks milk during ragweed season, his allergic load overcomes his tolerance or resistance causing him to develop allergy symptoms including wheezing, fatigue, irritability...

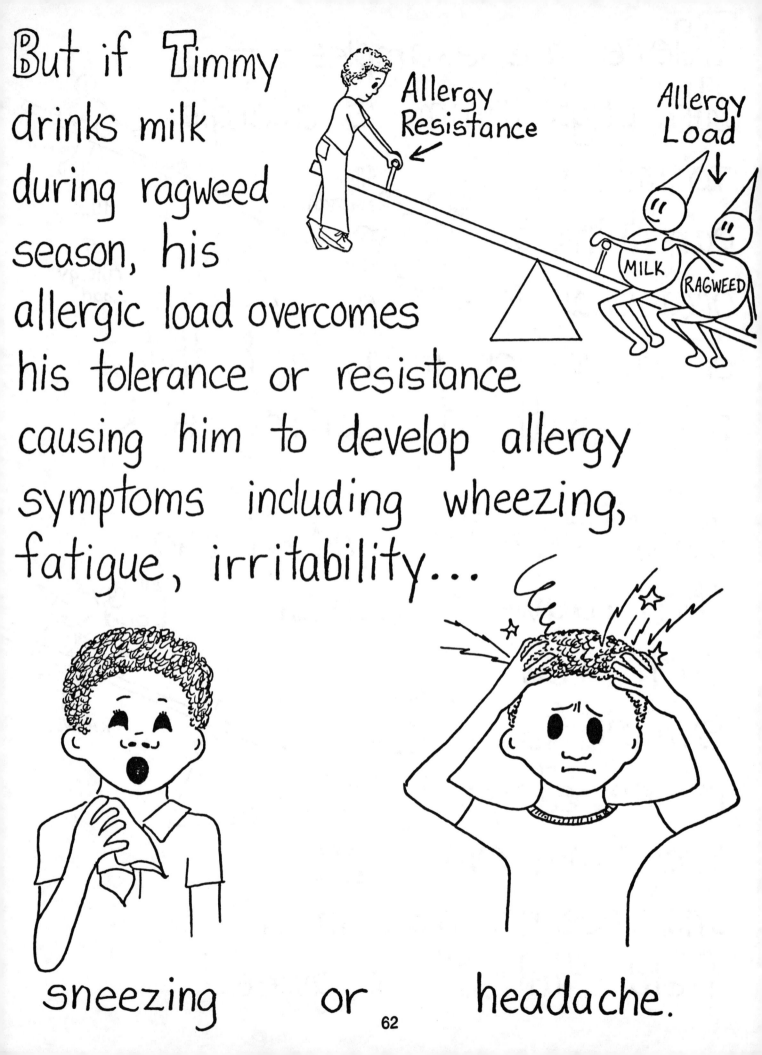

Allergy Resistance

Allergy Load

MILK

RAGWEED

sneezing   or   headache.

Timmy's allergy tolerance can also be overcome if...
he drinks alot of milk anytime during the year,
or...
if dust collects in his room, his pet sleeps on the foot of his bed and he's drinking milk.

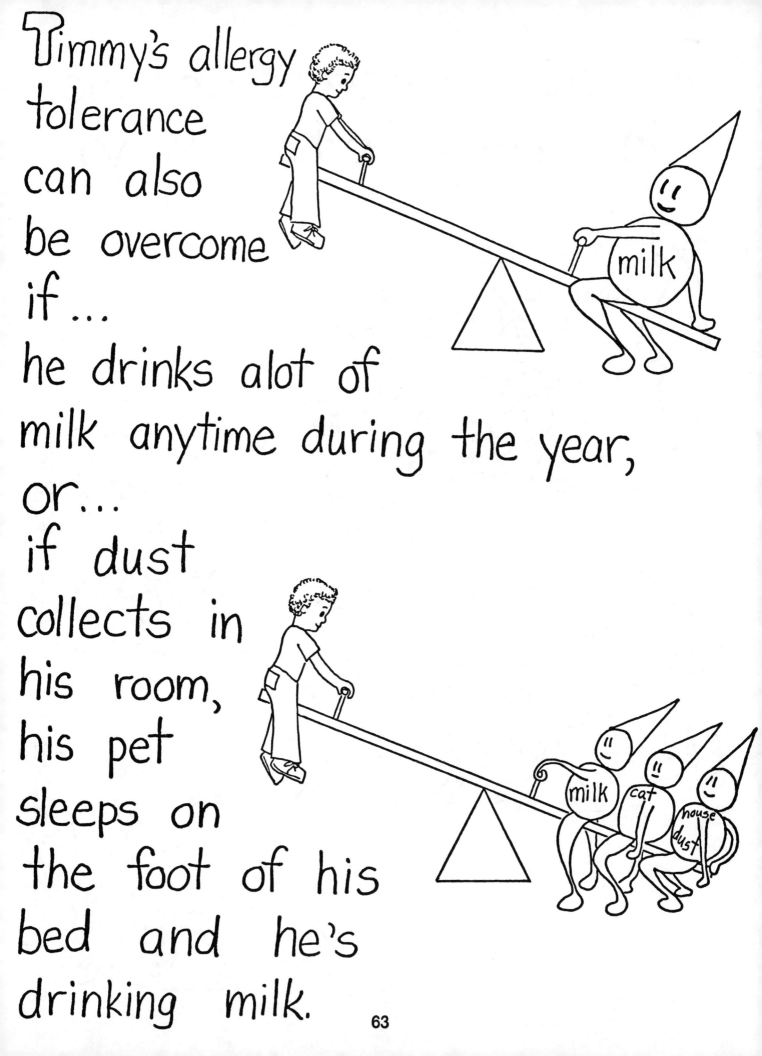

It can also be overcome in many other ways

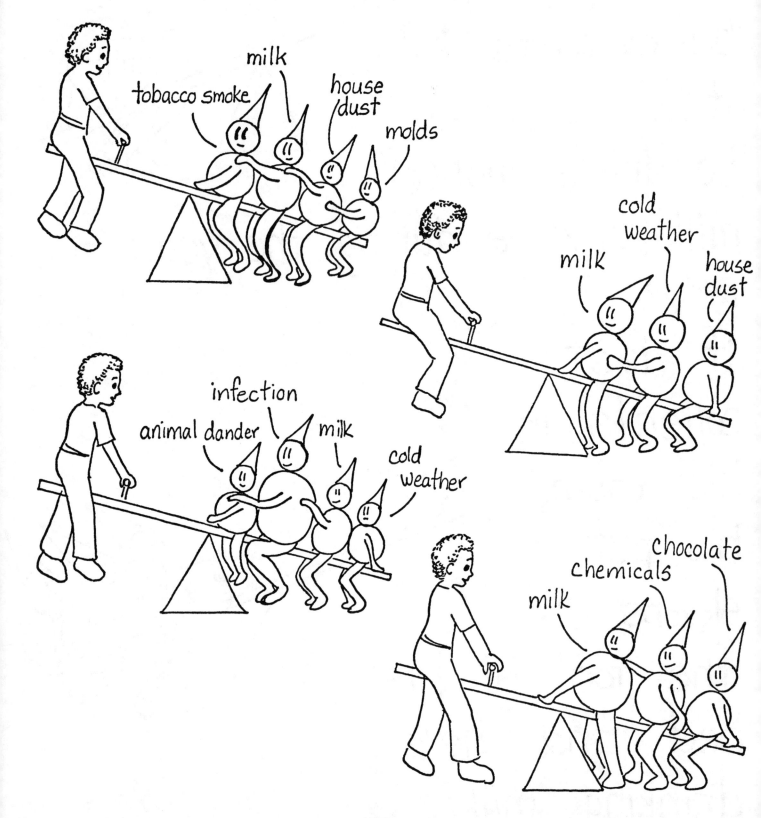

The best way to keep Timmy, your child, or any allergic child well is to: ①Find out which Allergy Gremlins give him trouble. ②Keep these Gremlins under control.

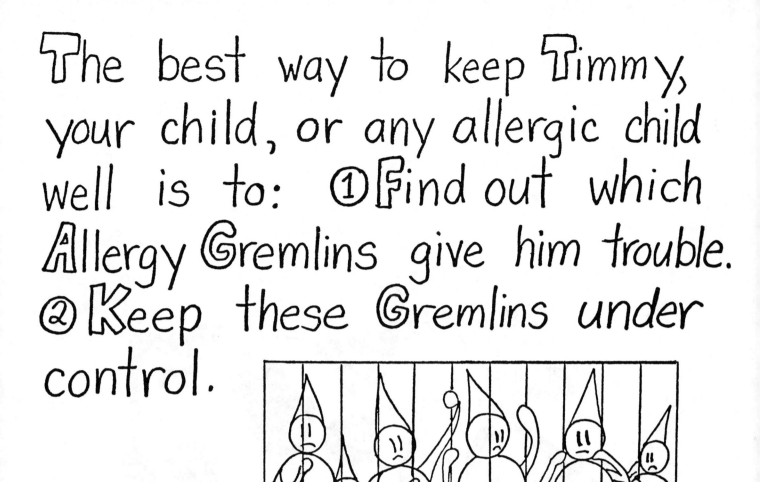

Gremlin Jail ⟶

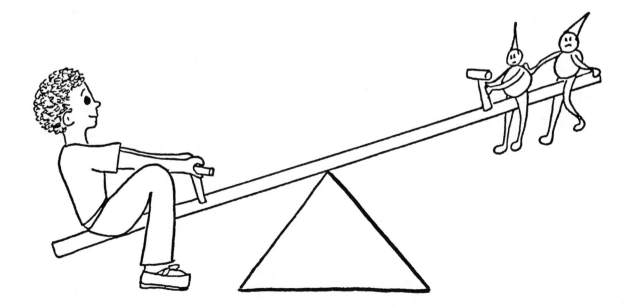

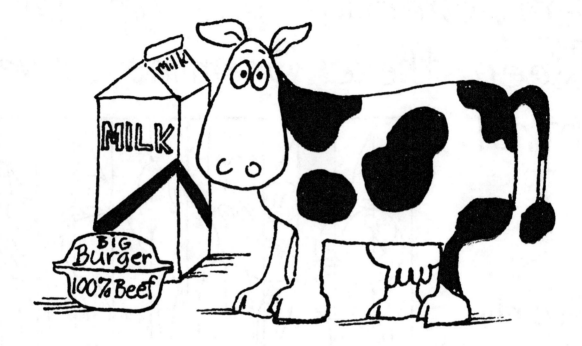

SUSIE'S COW'S MILK ALLERGY!

Susie's Cow's Milk Allergy

When Susie was an infant her mother nursed her and gave her only breast milk for many months.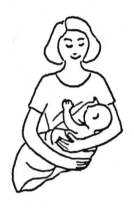

Susie thrived. She was happy and healthy. No colds, no skin rashes. And Susie rarely cried.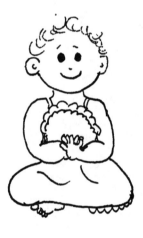

When Susie was nine months old, her mother weaned her and gave her cow's milk from a cup.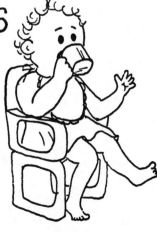

After a few weeks Susie developed a cough, cold and ear infection.

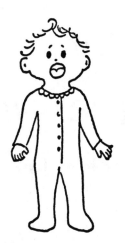

Although Susie's doctor prescribed several kinds of medicine, her symptoms persisted.

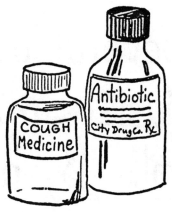

Then one day the doctor said, "Susie may be allergic to cow's milk. Don't give her milk for the next week and see what happens."

After three days
Susie was better.
And in six days
her symptoms vanished.

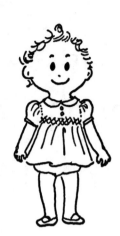

Several days later
Susie's mother gave her
milk. By bedtime her
nose was running and
she coughed all night.

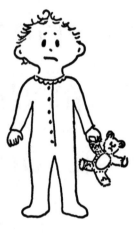

The milk was stopped.
In two days Susie's
"cold" dried up and
she felt fine.

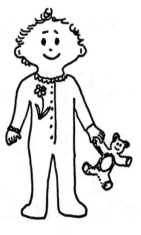

Susie drank no milk for six months. Then one day, her mother gave her milk and nothing happened.

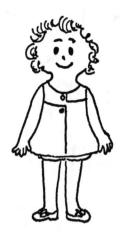

But when Susie drank milk five days in a row,

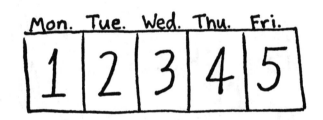

her cough, cold and irritability returned.

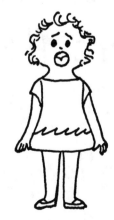

Susie again avoided milk (this time for a year) And now she can drink milk once a week and it doesn't bother her.

S	M	T	W	T	F	S
1	2	3	4	5	6	7
8	9	10	11	12	13	14
15	16	17	18	19	20	21
22	23	24	25	26	27	28
29	30	31				

↖ MILK DAY

Allergy to milk (or to any food) is like a fire... that dies down

Yet blowing on the embers (like eating a lot of the food) will cause the allergy to return.

72

ROTATED DIETS
OR
HOW PACO'S MOTHER
CONTROLS FOOD
ALLERGY GREMLINS

HOW PACO'S MOTHER CONTROLS FOOD ALLERGY GREMLINS

Paco's mother is smart. Very smart. She gives food allergy Gremlins "the run around" (in more ways than one!). And she succeeds because she rotates Paco's diet.

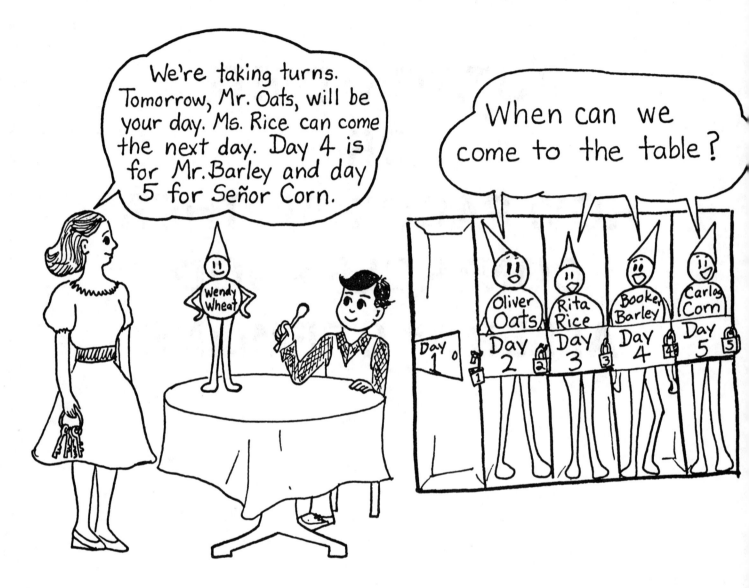

A rotated diet is a varied diet (and a carefully planned one, too.) Your child eats different foods each day. And he doesn't repeat a food more often than every 4 to 7 days.

Rotating your child's diet isn't easy. Yet if your child (or your family) is loaded with allergies, a rotated diet (or "rotary diversified diet") is an excellent method of preventing and treating allergies.

Rotated Diets

Day →	1	2	3	4	5
Meats	Beef	Chicken	Shrimp	Pork	Trout
Fruits	Orange	Banana	Pineapple	Grape	Apple
Vegetables	White potato	Sweet potato	Carrot	Squash	Peas, beans or other legumes
Grains	Wheat	Oats	Rice	Barley	Corn
Sweeteners	Cane sugar	Maple sugar	Beet sugar	Honey	Saccharin
Nuts	Pecan	Almond	Cashew	Brazil	Peanut
Fats + Oils	Butter	Safflower oil	Cottonseed oil	Sunflower oil	Corn oil
Miscellaneous	Milk	Egg	Chocolate	Carob	Coconut

*See page 76 for suggested menus for a 4 day rotated diet.

SAMPLE MENUS FOR A FOUR-DAY ROTATED DIET*

DAY ONE (Beef, citrus, white potato, wheat, cane sugar, pecans, dairy products & coffee.)

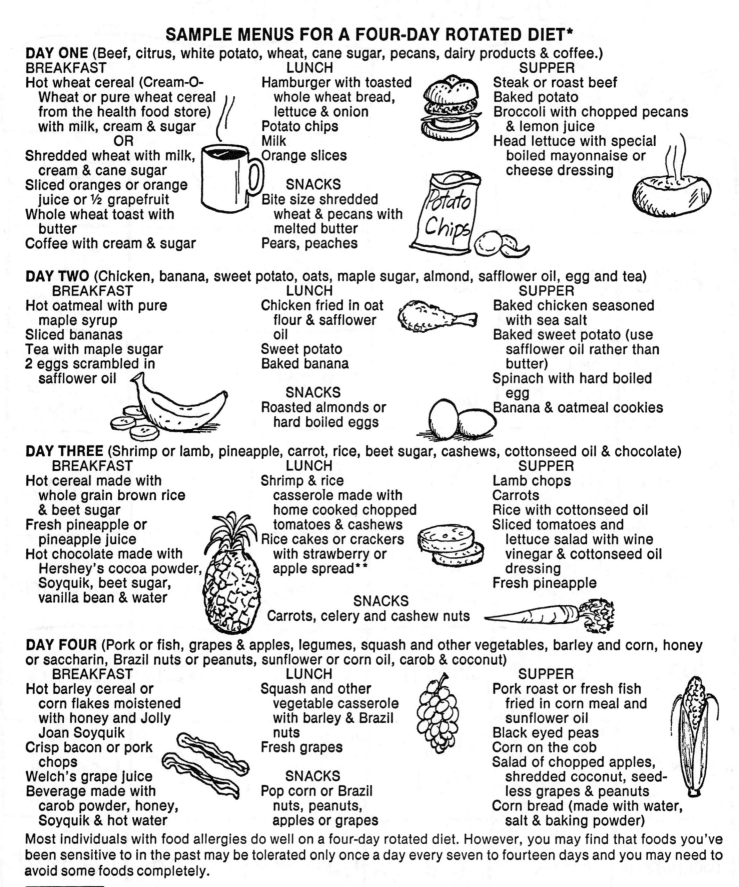

BREAKFAST

Hot wheat cereal (Cream-O-Wheat or pure wheat cereal from the health food store) with milk, cream & sugar
OR
Shredded wheat with milk, cream & cane sugar
Sliced oranges or orange juice or ½ grapefruit
Whole wheat toast with butter
Coffee with cream & sugar

LUNCH

Hamburger with toasted whole wheat bread, lettuce & onion
Potato chips
Milk
Orange slices

SNACKS
Bite size shredded wheat & pecans with melted butter
Pears, peaches

SUPPER

Steak or roast beef
Baked potato
Broccoli with chopped pecans & lemon juice
Head lettuce with special boiled mayonnaise or cheese dressing

DAY TWO (Chicken, banana, sweet potato, oats, maple sugar, almond, safflower oil, egg and tea)

BREAKFAST

Hot oatmeal with pure maple syrup
Sliced bananas
Tea with maple sugar
2 eggs scrambled in safflower oil

LUNCH

Chicken fried in oat flour & safflower oil
Sweet potato
Baked banana

SNACKS
Roasted almonds or hard boiled eggs

SUPPER

Baked chicken seasoned with sea salt
Baked sweet potato (use safflower oil rather than butter)
Spinach with hard boiled egg
Banana & oatmeal cookies

DAY THREE (Shrimp or lamb, pineapple, carrot, rice, beet sugar, cashews, cottonseed oil & chocolate)

BREAKFAST

Hot cereal made with whole grain brown rice & beet sugar
Fresh pineapple or pineapple juice
Hot chocolate made with Hershey's cocoa powder, Soyquik, beet sugar, vanilla bean & water

LUNCH

Shrimp & rice casserole made with home cooked chopped tomatoes & cashews
Rice cakes or crackers with strawberry or apple spread**

SNACKS
Carrots, celery and cashew nuts

SUPPER

Lamb chops
Carrots
Rice with cottonseed oil
Sliced tomatoes and lettuce salad with wine vinegar & cottonseed oil dressing
Fresh pineapple

DAY FOUR (Pork or fish, grapes & apples, legumes, squash and other vegetables, barley and corn, honey or saccharin, Brazil nuts or peanuts, sunflower or corn oil, carob & coconut)

BREAKFAST

Hot barley cereal or corn flakes moistened with honey and Jolly Joan Soyquik
Crisp bacon or pork chops
Welch's grape juice
Beverage made with carob powder, honey, Soyquik & hot water

LUNCH

Squash and other vegetable casserole with barley & Brazil nuts
Fresh grapes

SNACKS
Pop corn or Brazil nuts, peanuts, apples or grapes

SUPPER

Pork roast or fresh fish fried in corn meal and sunflower oil
Black eyed peas
Corn on the cob
Salad of chopped apples, shredded coconut, seedless grapes & peanuts
Corn bread (made with water, salt & baking powder)

Most individuals with food allergies do well on a four-day rotated diet. However, you may find that foods you've been sensitive to in the past may be tolerated only once a day every seven to fourteen days and you may need to avoid some foods completely.

---

*Individuals bothered by severe food allergies should eat each food at only one meal every 4 days.
**See food sources page 41.

YOU'LL NEED
TO KEEP A
DIARY

YOU'LL NEED TO KEEP A DIARY . . . .

To tell if your elimination diet makes a difference, you'll need to keep a diary. Buy an 8 x 10 inch notebook and use a new page each day. Begin the diary three days before you start eliminating foods. And continue it until the diet is completed.

Grade your symptoms:

       0—no symptoms
       1—mild symptoms
       2—moderate symptoms
       3—severe symptoms

Here are examples: If you sniff or your nose runs all the time, put "2" in the respiratory column for each period during the 24-hours.

If you complain of a bad headache on arising each day, which gradually disappears by lunch time, put a "3" in the headache column "before breakfast," a "2" in the morning column, and put a "0" in the headache column for the rest of the day.

At the bottom of the page, list the foods you eat each day.

By keeping this diary, you can usually tell which foods . . . if any . . . are causing your complaints.

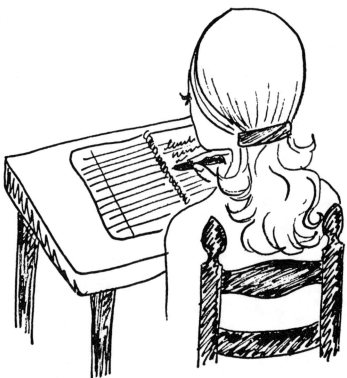

Symptom and Diet Diary

Time of Day → / Symptoms ↓	Before Breakfast	After Breakfast	After Lunch	After Supper	During Night
Tired or Drows					
Irritable or Overactive					
Headache					
Respirato (stuffy no cough, e					
Digestiv (bellyache nausea, e					
Urinary (bedwettin frequenc to)					
Other					

What you ate today ✍

Breakfast	Morning	Lunch	Afternoon	Supper	Evening

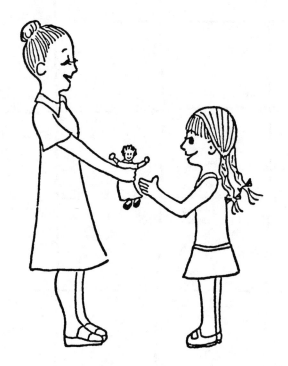

HELPING MARY
STAY ON HER DIET—
THE DIET GAME

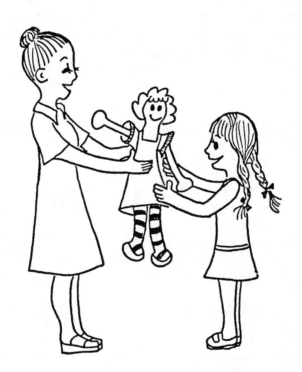

HELPING MARY STAY ON HER DIET

As Mary's mother thought about the diet, she said to herself, "Mary likes orange juice, frosted junkies and chocolate milk for breakfast; hot dogs and corn chips for lunch; and a cola after school. . . . She isn't going to like this diet . . . And I may run into trouble getting her to cooperate and not cheat."

Then Mary's mother had an idea. A bright idea. She said to her husband, "Mary loves games and prizes (and what child doesn't?), so I'll make a game out of the diet."

And here's what Mary's mother did: She made a chart and taped it to the door of the refrigerator. And she bought a box of stars for Mary to paste on the chart.

She told Mary about the diet, saying, "Mama is going to buy extra special foods for you to eat for the next two weeks. And we're going to play 'the diet game'."

"What kind of game is that?" asked Mary. "And how can I win prizes?"

Mama replied, "By eating foods . . . like a hamburger patty and french fries for breakfast; bananas, peanut butter and rice crackers for lunch; pineapple juice, raisins and pecans for a snack. If you eat only the foods on your diet, you'll earn six stars a day to paste on your chart. And each night at bedtime, you'll win a prize."

"Goody, goody," said Mary.

"And at the end of about two weeks," continued mama, "if you stay on your diet and don't cheat, you'll win a *big* prize."

Mary's Diet Game Chart

	Monday	Tuesday	Wednesday	Thursday	Friday	Saturday	Sunday
Breakfast	☆	☆					
Morning	☆	☆					
Lunch	☆	☆					
Afternoon	☆	☆					
Supper	☆	☆					
Evening	☆	☆					

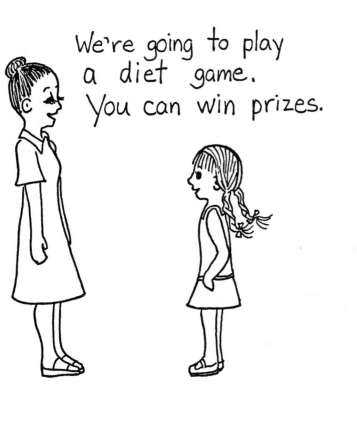

We're going to play
a diet game.
You can win prizes.

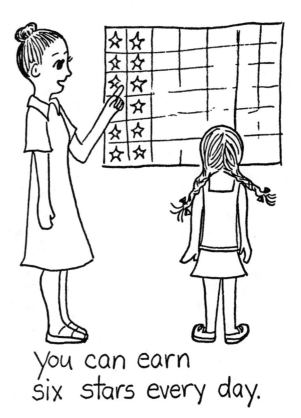

You can earn
six stars every day.

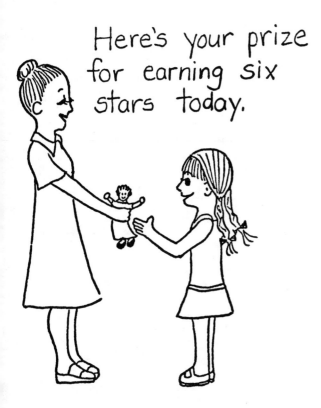

Here's your prize
for earning six
stars today.

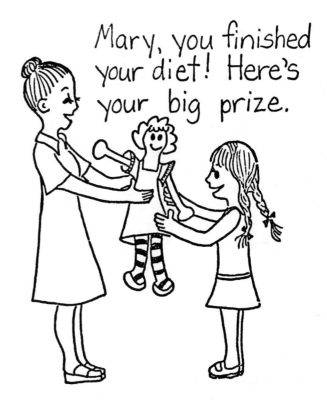

Mary, you finished
your diet! Here's
your big prize.

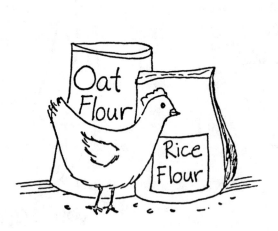

RECIPES
FOR ELIMINATION DIET A

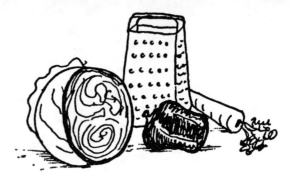

COLE SLAW

shredded cabbage
grated carrots
minced green pepper or pineapple
special boiled mayonnaise

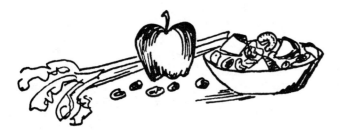

CHICKEN-RICE SOUP

6 cups chicken stock (water in which
  chicken has been stewed)
½ cup brown rice (raw)
⅓ cup onion, diced
⅓ cup celery
2 tablespoons safflower oil
1 cup cooked chicken diced
Salt
2 tablespoons chopped parsley

Heat chicken stock to boiling. Add rice and simmer 35 minutes.

Saute onion and celery in oil for about 5 minutes and add to soup. Add chicken, correct seasoning and just before serving, add parsley.

Yield: Approximately 6 servings.

WALDORF SALAD

1 apple, cored and chopped
celery, chopped
1 tablespoon chopped pecans
1 tablespoon raisins
special boiled mayonnaise

Combine apple, raisins, pecans, and celery. Mix lightly with boiled mayonnaise until all pieces are coated. Chill.

SPECIAL BOILED MAYONNAISE

1½ tablespoons potato starch flour
½ teaspoon salt
¼ teaspoon dry mustard
1-3 tablespoons wine or apple cider vinegar *
¼ cup cold water
¾ cup boiling water
3 tablespoons wine or apple cider vinegar**
½ cup safflower or sunflower oil
salt and pepper

Combine the potato starch, salt, dry mustard, and wine (or apple cider vinegar) in a saucepan and stir to a smooth paste with the ¼ cup cold water. Add the boiling water and cook only until mixture is clear. Remove from heat and cool to lukewarm. Add vinegar and oil, beating constantly. Season with salt and pepper. Makes 1¼ cup.

---

*The amount of vinegar added will depend on taste.
**Added after cooking.

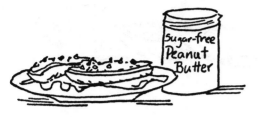

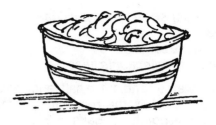

PEANUT BUTTER AND BANANA SALAD

Slice a banana into fourths. Coat with a layer of peanut butter. Sprinkle chopped pecans over the top. Serve on lettuce leaf.

CHICKEN SALAD

cooked chicken, diced
celery, chopped
salt and pepper to taste
special boiled mayonnaise

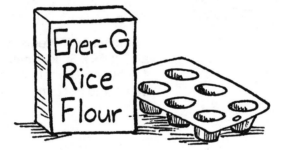

RICE MUFFINS

1½ cups rice flour
½ teaspoon salt
2 teaspoons baking powder*
¼ teaspoon soda
4 tablespoons oil (sunflower or safflower)
1 tablespoon honey
3 tablespoons apricot puree
1 cup water or Soyquik

Place all ingredients in a mixing bowl in above order, and stir until batter is smooth. Spoon batter into greased muffin tin and bake at 350° for 15-20 minutes.
Makes 12 muffins.

---

*Use Cellu brand baking powder since most baking powders contain corn.

CANDIED SWEET POTATOES

3 or 4 medium-sized sweet potatoes
1 cup honey
2 tablespoons safflower oil
¼ cup water or pineapple juice

Peel the potatoes and cut in half lengthwise. Arrange in baking dish. Mix the remaining ingredients and pour over the potatoes. Bake at 375 degrees for 50 minutes.

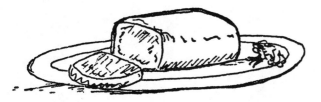

SPECIAL MEAT LOAF

2 lbs. ground beef
⅓ cup minute tapioca
⅓ cup onion, finely chopped
1½ teaspoons salt
¼ teaspoon pepper
1½ canned tomatoes, mashed

Combine all ingredients, mixing well. Then pack into a 9″ x 5″ x 3″ loaf pan. Bake at 350 degrees for 1 to 1¼ hours. Unmold on serving platter and slice. May be served hot or cold. Makes 6 to 8 servings.

OVEN BAKED CHICKEN

Preheat oven to 350°

8-10 pieces of chicken
½ cup rice flour (Jolly Joan)
½ cup oat flour (Jolly Joan)
¾ teaspoon salt
1/8 teaspoon pepper

Mix flour and seasoning and put in paper bag. Put 2 or 3 pieces of chicken in bag and shake to coat. Continue until all pieces are coated.
Place chicken, skin side up, in oiled pan. Brush each piece lightly with safflower oil. Bake in oven for one hour or until chicken is nicely browned and tender.
GRAVY: Strain pan liquid into saucepan: Dissolve 1 tablespoon oat flour and 1 tablespoon arrowroot powder in ½ cup hot water. Add to pan liquid, stirring, and bring to a boil. Add more chicken stock or water to make desired consistency.

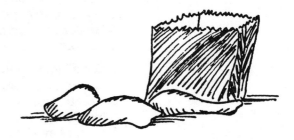

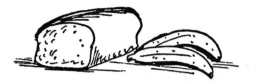

BANANA BREAD*

1½ cups brown rice flour
2 teaspoons Cellu brand baking powder
pinch of salt, cinnamon, nutmeg and cloves
2 ripe bananas
5 tablespoons Safflower oil
½ cup plus 2 tablespoons honey
2 tablespoons egg substitute
⅔ cups chopped walnuts.

Sift the flour, baking powder and spices together. Mash the bananas and blend with the oil, honey and egg substitute. Slowly add dry mix to oil mixture. Blend well. Add nuts. Pour into well greased bread pan and bake at 350° for 50 to 60 minutes.

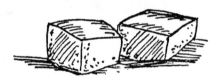

PINEAPPLE NUT BREAD*

2¼ cups rolled oats (put in blender to make a meal)
4 teaspoons Cellu-brand baking powder
¼ teaspoon soda
¾ teaspoon salt
¾ cup honey
¾ cup chopped nuts
2 tablespoons safflower oil
½ cup pineapple juice

Directions:

1. Preheat oven to 350°. Grease 9″ x 5″ loaf pan.
2. Mix dry ingredients thoroughly.
3. Add nuts, oil and pineapple juice.
4. Stir until dry ingredients are well moistened.
5. Pour into pan.
6. Bake 60-minutes or until firm to touch.
7. To prevent the top of loaf from cracking, cover with foil during first 20-minutes of baking time. Makes 1 loaf.

RICE-OAT MUFFINS

1 cup rolled oats (ground)
¾ cup rice flour
2 tablespoons Cellu brand baking powder
1 teaspoon salt
1 teaspoon cinnamon
¼ cup honey
½ cup raisins
¼ cup safflower oil
1 cup water

Directions:

1. Preheat oven to 425°.
2. Grease muffin tins.
3. Mix dry ingredients thoroughly.
4. Add raisins, water and oil. Mix well.
5. Fill muffin tins about ⅔ full.
6. Bake 20 minutes or until lightly browned. Makes 12 muffins.

GINGERBREAD

1 cup honey
½ cup boiling water
2¼ cups rice flour (or 1-1/8 cups rice flour and 1-1/8 cups potato flour)
1 teaspoon baking powder
½ teaspoon soda
1½ teaspoons ginger
½ teaspoon salt
4 tablespoons melted Willow Run margarine
1 teaspoon vanilla

Mix honey and boiling water. Sift dry ingredients together. Add the dry ingredients to the honey mixture. Add the melted margarine and vanilla. Beat well. Pour into a greased baking pan and bake at 350 degrees for 30 minutes.

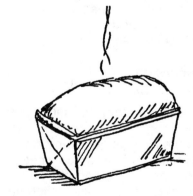

*You'll obtain additional recipes for making bread on the outside of boxes of Jolly Joan & Ener-G Brown Rice & White Rice Baking Mix.

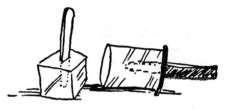

POPSICLES

Take apple juice, pineapple juice, or pure Welch's grape juice and pour into a special mold or ice-cube tray for "homemade" popsicles.

PANCAKES

½ cup rice flour
¾ cup oats (whole grain or
   quick cooking)
1 tablespoon Cellu baking powder
¼ teaspoon baking soda
2 tablespoons honey
2 tablespoons safflower or soy oil
½ teaspoon salt
3 tablespoons apricot puree
   (to replace egg)
½ cup Soyquik

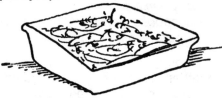

Place ¾ cup of oats in blender container; cover & blend until the oats are like a fine meal, then add formula, oil, honey & apricot puree. Beat mixture until smooth. Drop by tablespoons on lightly greased griddle set at medium low to low heat. Let pancakes cook until fairly well set, then turn carefully. Serve with honey or maple syrup.

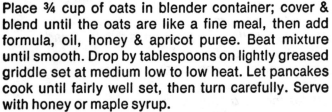

APPLE CRISP

4 cups sliced cooking apples
1 cup Quaker or Mother's Oats
   (quick or old fashioned, uncooked)
½ cup honey
1 teaspoon cinnamon
¼ cup safflower or sunflower oil

Drop apple slices in water with 2 tablespoons of wine or apple cider vinegar to keep apples from browning. Then place apples in shallow baking dish. Mix oil and oats in a small mixing bowl at low speed until it has the texture of corn meal. Add cinnamon; then add honey to this mixture. Sprinkle crumb mixture over apples. Bake in pre-heated moderate oven (375 degrees) for 30-minutes or until apples are tender. Makes 6 servings.

HONEY BARS

½ cup Willow Run margarine
1 cup honey
2 cups Quaker rolled oats
¼ teaspoon salt
1 teaspoon baking powder
¼ teaspoon soda
1 teaspoon vanilla

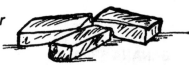

Combine margarine and honey in a saucepan; cook and stir until margarine melts. Stir in remaining ingredients. Mix well. Pour into greased 8" x 8" x 2" baking pan. Bake in 350 degree oven for 20 to 25 minutes. Cool; cut into bars. Makes 2 dozen.

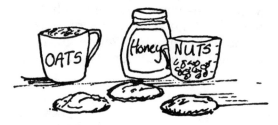

OATMEAL COOKIES

1 cup quick-cooking rolled oats
½ cup ground nuts
½ cup chopped nuts
¼ cup safflower or soy oil
¼ cup honey
¼ teaspoon baking powder
¼ teaspoon baking soda
½ teaspoon salt
1 teaspoon vanilla (pure)
¼ cup quick cooking rolled oats

Place ½ cup of the oats in blender container; cover & blend till oats are like a fine meal. Repeat with another ½ cup oats. Place ½ cup nuts in blender container and blend until coarse meal. Combine blended oats, ground nuts, chopped nuts, baking powder and soda and salt. Stir in safflower or soy oil, honey & vanilla. Sprinkle foil or wax paper with ¼ cup oats. Roll dough in oats to cover surface of dough. Roll dough to a 10 inch circle about 1/8" thick. Cut into 8 wedges. Place on a lightly greased baking sheet. Lift foil or wax paper and invert quickly onto baking sheet to avoid tearing the dough. Bake at 325° for 12-15 min. Turn off heat and open oven door. Leave in oven until firm & crisp, 4-5 min.

THE
CHEMICAL PROBLEM

THE CHEMICAL PROBLEM*

Let's suppose you follow the instructions in this book and you improve. Yet, you continue to experience symptoms. And such symptoms are caused by something you're eating.

In this situation, you'll have to search further. And you may find you are bothered by sensitivity to chemicals in food and food containers (including cans, plastic wrappings and boxes). Many chemical contaminants in foods are derived from petro-chemicals and coal tars. Others come from antibiotics and insecticides.

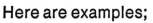

Here are examples;

Bananas picked green are usually exposed to a petroleum-derived gas, ethylene. So are apples, pears, oranges and tomatoes.

Chickens may contain antibiotics, hormones and other chemicals. baked chicken

Sugar is usually treated with chemicals of various sorts during processing.

Peelings on fresh fruits and vegetables often contain insecticide and herbicide residues. They also may be coated with mineral oils and waxes to give them an attractive shine.

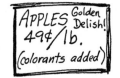

APPLES Golden
Delish!
49¢/lb.
(colorants added)

French fried potatoes may be treated with chemicals to prevent discoloration. white potato

Beef and pork may contain chemicals and hormones of various sorts. Some are administered to the animal before slaughtering; some are added to the meat as preservatives.

pork chop

Tap water often contains chemicals from a variety of sources. These include insecticides and weed killers which remain in the water in spite of purification and filtration; chemicals added to the water including fluorine and chlorine; chemicals picked up from plastic pipes or copper pipes.

Tracking down a hidden chemical allergy is even more difficult than tracking down hidden food allergy. However, it can be done. Here are suggestions that may help you.

---

*Adapted from material prepared by Dr. Theron Randolph

1. Use well, spring or distilled water.

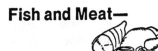

2. Obtain foods from organic sources. (Some farmers, growers and packers specialize in raising and producing foods which are as free of chemical contamination as humanly possible. You'll find a list of some of them in the Food Sources section.)

3. Use no canned or packaged food in diets to determine chemical sensitivity.

4. If you use commercial foods, purchase those in glass containers. (Avoid canned foods and those wrapped in plastic.)

5. Use glass jars or containers (rather than plastic) to store foods in your own refrigerator.

6. Purchase meats, fruits, vegetables, grains from growers in your area who use organic farming methods. (You can obtain such a list of growers by writing to PREVENTION MAGAZINE, Emmaus, Pennsylvania.)

7. Foods less apt to be chemically contaminated include:

Fish and Meat— Seafood and meat from which the fat has been stripped prior to cooking.

Vegetables— Potato (undyed and home-peeled), turnips, egg plant, tomato (if field ripened), carrots (but not bagged in plastic), squash, okra, green peas and green beans.

Fruit— Cantaloupe, watermelon, fresh pineapple

Miscellaneous— Nuts (in shell only), Brazil nuts, coconut, walnut, hickory nut, pecan, filbert, hazel nut.

Sweetening agents— Honey, maple and sorghum

Fats and Oils— Olive, cottonseed, peanut, soy, coconut, safflower, sunflower

Postscript

Allergy is a "peculiar" branch of medicine. Perhaps its main peculiarity is that doctors . . . including allergists . . . continue to disagree among themselves about the definition of the term "allergy." The crux of the controversy involves mainly food allergy, more especially what has been termed "hidden" or "delayed onset" food allergy.

One group of physicians feels the term "allergy" should include only those disorders which can be demonstrated by presently available immunologic methods . . . including the allergy scratch test.

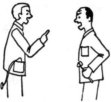

Many of the these physicians work in departments of immunologic research in university medical centers. Yet other physicians who hold similar views are in practice. Representative of this point of view are Dr. Richard S. Farr and Dr. Charles May of the National Jewish Hospital and Research Center in Denver, Colorado.

In discussing the controversy, these physicians say, in effect, "To make a diagnosis of allergy, you must be able to explain it on the basis of known immunologic mechanisms. This is a very stringent definition because it *insists* that the immunologic mechanism be identified as causing or contributing to the cause of illness. And in identifying such an immunologic mechanism, the vast majority of practicing physicians must rely upon the skin test." (Other immunologists feel that the RAST (radioallergosorbent test) or other immunologic tests must be positive to show that a "truly allergic disorder" exists.)

However, such physicians present only one side of this controversy. Here's the other side; here's how many other physicians look on allergy:

Some 50 years ago, the late Dr. Albert Rowe, Sr. of Oakland, California noted that many of his patients showed adverse reactions to common foods, especially milk, egg and the cereal grains. In some of his patients, these adverse reactions would produce symptoms of sneezing, wheezing or itching; yet in other patients, these reactions would cause fatigue, irritability, headache, abdominal pain, muscle aching and bladder symptoms. Because these reactions were caused by specific hypersensitivity to foods, Dr. Rowe used the term "food allergy" to apply to these reactions.

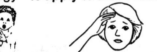

After studying thousands of food sensitive patients, Dr. Rowe said, in effect, "Unsuspected food allergy causes more allergic reactions than inhalant and drug allergies. In fact, most people, at some time in their lives, suffer in varying degrees from allergy to foods. To detect the presence of food allergy, the diet must be manipulated. *The usual allergy skin test is not an accurate way of determining the presence or absence of food allergy. What's more, too much reliance on the allergy scratch test is one of the main causes of confusion in the field of allergy today."*

Physicians holding this sort of view of food allergy who have been working both in allergy research and practice during the last two decades include Doctors James Breneman, Joe Bullock, William Deamer, John Gerrard, Jerome Glaser, James O'Shea, Theron Randolph, Doris Rapp, Albert Rowe, Jr., Douglas Sandberg, Frederic Speer, Robert Stroud and many, many others.

In commenting on this controversy, Dr. Speer of the University of Kansas said, in effect, "I'm sure that anybody will agree that there is a need to discuss just what the clinician is to include under the term 'allergy' . . . I know there are allergists who refuse to recognize allergy in the absence of positive laboratory findings and skin tests . . . But I feel if they continue to hold this sort of position, a vast amount of human suffering will go unrelieved . . . I prefer to use the term 'allergy' broadly in a clinical sense."

Dr. William C. Deamer of the University of California commented, saying, in effect, "It would certainly clear up some of the confusion among both doctors and patients if we had a laboratory test to identify delayed onset food allergy. But we don't. Yet I do not believe we need to sit back and wait for such a laboratory test. Instead, we can identify and successfully treat the patient with systemic food allergy by using elimination diets."

Because of this controversy among respected physicians, the patient is often "caught in the middle" and confused by their differing opinions over what should and should not be called "food allergy."

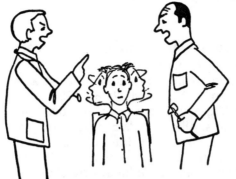

Recently, a professor of English at a Tennessee college commented, "For years I was bothered by a stuffy nose, fatigue, irritability and headaches. I consulted many physicians, including an allergist, in my effort to obtain help. All my tests were negative and my physicians said, 'You don't have an allergy.' Then, someone suggested that I do an elimination diet. I did, and my symptoms vanished. And they returned when I drank milk or ate corn.

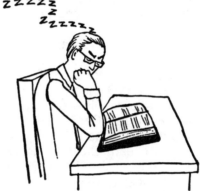

Now, after having avoided these foods for three years, I rarely suffer from a headache, my energy level has improved dramatically, and nasal congestion rarely bothers me."

And he continued, "I couldn't care less whether you doctors call my condition 'allergy' or whether you call it by some other term. *The important thing is that I found that foods I was eating every day were causing my symptoms and now that I avoid them, my health has improved a hundred percent.*"

If you're bothered by symptoms like those of the college professor, you can easily determine whether they're related to common foods by trying a carefully designed and executed elimination diet. And you don't need to wait for scientists to explain the mechanisms involved.

Moreover, the physician who prescribes such diets can feel comfortable in doing so because he'll be following the examples set by Doctors Jenner, Lind, Semmelweiss, and many others during the previous centuries (Jenner innoculated people with cowpox and prevented smallpox; Lind gave British sailors limes and kept them from dying of scurvy; Semmelweiss made medical students in Vienna wash their hands before doing pelvic examinations and prevented the spread of fatal streptococcal "childbed fever"). *These three physicians and many others used these safe therapies which helped their patients because they knew the therapies worked, rather than waiting for "scientific proof" which was delayed for decades or even centuries.*

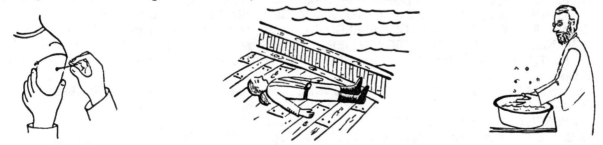

Over 200 scientific articles on the subject of hidden or delayed onset food allergy have been published in the medical literature during the past 75 years. In addition, the subject has been dealt with in over 40 books written for both professionals and non-professionals. Listed on the following page are a few of these references.

References from the medical literature of interest mainly to professionals:

Hare, F.: THE FOOD FACTOR IN DISEASE. London, Longmans, Green & Co., 1905, Vols. I, II.

Shannon, W.R.: Neuropathic Manifestations In Infants and Children as a Result of Anaphylactic Reactions to Foods Contained in Their Dietary. Am. J. Dis. Child., 24:89, 1922.

Rowe, A.H., Sr.: Allergic Toxemia and Migraine Due to Food Allergy. Calif. West. Med, 33:785, 1930.

Rowe, A.H., Sr.: Chronic Ulcerative Colitis, Allergy in its Etiology. Ann. Int. Med., 17:83, 1942.

Rinkel, H.J.: Food Allergy: The Role of Food Allergy in Internal Medicine. Annals of Allergy, 2:115, 1944.

Rowe, A.H.: Elimination Diets and the Patient's Allergies. Philadelphia, Lea & Febiger, 1944.

Randolph, T.G.: Allergy as a Causative Factor of Fatigue, Irritability, and Behavior Problems in Children. J. Pediat., 32:266, 1948.

Davison, H.M.: Allergy of the Nervous System. Quart. Rev. Allerg., 6:157, 1952.

Speer, F.: The Allergic Tension-Fatigue Syndrome. Ped. Clin. N. Amer., 1:1029, 1954.

Breneman, J.C.: Allergic Cystitis: The Cause of Nocturnal Enuresis. GP, 20:84, 1959.

Crook, W.G., Harrison, W.W., Crawford, S.E., and Emerson, B.S.: Systemic Manifestations Due to Allergy. Report of Fifty Patients and a Review of the Literature on the Subject. Pediat., 27:790, 1961.

Rinkel, H.J., Lee, C.H., Brown, D.W., Willoughby, J.W., and Williams, J.M.: The Diagnosis of Food Allergy. Arch of Otolaryngology, 79:71, 1964.

Bullock, J.D., Deamer, W.C., Frick, O.L., Crisp, J.R., III, Galant, S.P., and Ziering, W.H.: Recurrent Abdominal Pain. (Letters) Pediatrics, 46:969, 1970.

Kemp, J.P.: Recurrent Abdominal Pain. (Letters) Pediatrics, 46:969, 1970.

Deamer, W.C.: Pediatric Allergy: Some Impressions Gained Over a 37-Year Period. Pediatrics, 48:930, 1971.

Campbell, M.B.: Neurologic Manifestations of Allergic Disease. Ann. Allerg., 31:485, 1973.

Sandberg, D.H.: Recurrent Abdominal Pain: Recurrent Controversy. (Letters) Pediatrics, 51:307, 1973.

Miller, J.B.: A Double-Blind Study of Food Extract Injection Therapy: Ann. of Allerg., 38:185, 1977.

Rapp, D.J.: Does Diet Affect Hyperactivity? J. of Learn. Disabil., 11:383, 1978.

Rapp, D.J.: Food Allergy Treatment for Hyperkinesis. J. of Learn. Disabil., 1978.

Crook, W.G.: Adverse Reactions to Food Can Cause Hyperkinesis. (Letters) Am. J. Dis. Child., 132:819, 1978.

Grant, E.C.G.: Food Allergies and Migraine. Lancet, 1:966, 1979.

Deamer, W.C., Gerrard, J.W., and Speer, F.: Cow's Milk Allergy: J. of Fam. Prac., 9:223, 1979.

Crook, W.G.: What Is Scientific Proof? Pediatrics, 65:638, 1980.

Ogle, K., and Bullock, J.D.: Children with Allergic Rhinitis and/or Bronchial Asthma Treated with Elimination Diet: A Five-Year Follow-Up. Ann. Allergy, 44:273, 1980.

Crook, W.G.: Can What Child Eats Make Him Dull, Stupid or Hyperactive? J. of Learn. Disabil., 13:281 1980.

Contemporary books on hidden food allergy of interest to both professionals and non-professionals:

Gerrard, J.W.: UNDERSTANDING ALLERGIES. Springfield, Ill., Charles C. Thomas, 1973.

Mackarness, R.: EATING DANGEROUSLY. New York, Harcourt Brace Jovanovich, 1976.

Mackarness, R.: NOT ALL IN THE MIND. London, Pan Books, Ltd., 1976.

Oski, F.: DON'T DRINK YOUR MILK. New York, Wyden Books, 1977.

Crook, W.G.: CAN YOUR CHILD READ? IS HE HYPERACTIVE? Jackson, Tenn. Professional Books, 1977.

Crook, W.G.: ARE YOU ALLERGIC? (former title: YOUR ALLERGIC CHILD, Williams & Wilkins), Jackson, Tenn., Professional Books, 1978 (revised).

Rapp, D.J.: ALLERGIES AND THE HYPERACTIVE CHILD. New York, Sovereign Books, 1980.

Forman, R.: HOW TO CONTROL YOUR ALLERGIES. New York, Larchmont Books, 1979.

McGee, C.: HOW TO SURVIVE MODERN TECHNOLOGY. Alamo, California, Ecology Press, 1979.

Golos, N., and Golbitz, F.G.: COPING WITH YOUR ALLERGIES. New York, Simon & Schuster, 1979.

Mandell, M.: DR. MANDELL'S FIVE DAY ALLERGY RELIEF SYSTEM. New York, Crowell, 1979.

Stevens, L.J.: HOW TO IMPROVE YOUR CHILD'S BEHAVIOR THROUGH DIET. Garden City, New York, Doubleday & Company, 1979.

Sheinkin, D., Schacter, M., and Hutton, R.: THE FOOD CONNECTION. Indianapolis, Bobbs-Merrill, 1979.

Rapp, D.J.: ALLERGIES AND YOUR FAMILY. New York, Sterling Publishing Company, 1980.

Speer, F.: FOOD ALLERGY, Littleton, Mass., PSG Publishing Co., Inc. 1978

Breneman, J. C.: BASICS OF FOOD ALLERGY. Chas. C. Thomas, Springfield, 1978.

Randolph, T.G. and Moss, R.: An Alternative Approach to Allergies. New York, Harper & Row, 1980.

Many of these books may be obtained from your local bookstore or health food store. Or they can be ordered from: Dickey Enterprises, 109 W. Olive St., Fort Collins, Colorado 80521; or from Aurora Book Companions, Box 5852, Denver, Colorado 80217